You Are the Future of Acupuncture and Oriental Medicine.

- ■ Will acupuncture be a subset of medical practice for MDs only?
- ■ Will it be a supporting health care practice equivalent to physiotherapy?
- ■ Will it be a medical alternative equal to western medicine?
- ■ Can you conceive of it being a major form of health care for everyone?
- ■ Could it ever replace western medicine?
- ■ Or, could it die out?

The Future of acupuncture and oriental medicine is in your hands...

May this book guide you along your path.

How To Start And Successfully Manage Your Practice

by
Cynthia Flint Bestani
with Dr. Peter G. Fernandez

FOCUS PRACTICE MANAGEMENT PUBLICATIONS

Volume I: The Acupuncture Practice Management Guide: *How to Start and Successfully Manage Your Practice,* Revised edition. 1992, 1996, 1997, 1998. Copyright ©1988, ©1992, ©1996, ©1997, ©1998 by Cynthia Flint Bestani.

The Acupuncture Practice Management Guide: Volumes I-IV, ©.1986
The Acupuncture Practice Management Guide: Volume I: How to Start and Successfully Operate Your Practice, Copyright ©1987, How to Start and Successfully Manage Your Practice ©1992, ©1996, ©1997, ©1998 by Cynthia Flint Bestani.

Published by Focus Practice Management Publications, by special arrangements with the primary author. Communication with the publisher should be directed to 1 (800) 800-3139

ISBN: 0-944876-22-6 (Volume I)
ISBN: 0-944876-26-9 (Set of Volumes I-IV)

Printed in the U.S.A.

THE ACUPUNCTURE
PRACTICE MANAGEMENT GUIDE SERIES

About the Authors

Cynthia Flint Bestani has been a practice management consultant since 1984 primarily in the allied health professional field. She specializes in acupuncture practice management and has instructed at the former California Acupuncture College in Santa Barbara, California. She has written numerous books and pamphlets specifically for the acupuncture field as well as recorded audio tapes on practice management. She has spoken on practice management at acupuncture conferences at the state, national, and international levels. If you wish to be notified of future practice management publications or wish a private phone consultation, she may be contacted through Focus Practice Management Publications Distribution at 1 (800) 800-3139.

Dr. Peter G. Fernandez is listed as coauthor by his request and by the primary author's delight. He has provided substantial authority to what is offered in this book through the use of proven ideas and materials which both consultants have found work. Dr. Fernandez is one of the foremost respected consultants in the field of practice management for chiropractors and has written numerous books. His organization Fernandez Discipline holds seminars throughout the United States, primarily for chiropractors. Since increasing numbers of chiropractors are receiving acupuncture training, his program would have benefit to acupuncturists as well. His address is: Fernandez Discipline, 7777 131st. St. North, Suite 15, Seminole, Florida 33776. Phone number: (813) 392-0822.

Dedication

This series of books is dedicated to you whose purpose is healing through acupuncture — with all our best desires and intentions for your success.

It is for all those who love to practice acupuncture.

It is for those who are willing to open the door of success and well-being.

This fourth book is a tribute to effective choice — in how YOU want to communicate your practice.

THE ACUPUNCTURE PRACTICE MANAGEMENT GUIDE SERIES IS:
Dedicated to those who will integrate the art of healing with clear business practice.

Dedicated to setting a foundation and standard of professionalism in the practice of acupuncture.

Dedicated to increase the respect for acupuncture practitioners within the healing professions and in the public eye.

Dedicated to the creation of health care practices in which people can be at ease with acupuncture care and spread its benefits to others.

Dedicated to all those who may experience the healing benefits which acupuncture offers because of you.

Notice

This publication is designed to provide accurate and authoritative information in regard to the subject matter covered. It is sold with the understanding that the authors and the publisher are not a substitute for legal and accounting advice, and are not responsible for misspellings, omissions, or incorrect numbers.

Printed practice forms on excellent quality paper, as well as customized services, are available and can be ordered through Focus Practice Management Publications.

The manual is intended for direct use by the acupuncturist who wants to set-up a practice or expand his or her established practice.

Permission is granted for material use 1) by teachers only within the context of the business management classes of state accredited acupuncture colleges and 2) as a textbook for students within the business management classes of state accredited acupuncture colleges.

Acknowledgments

I am deeply grateful to the many health practitioners, office staff, friends, and other practice management consultants who have inspired me to bring this manual into being. I would particularly acknowledge the work forerun by Dr. Peter Fernandez and Dr. James Parker in chiropractic who have added much to the success of what could be presented here; Dr. Archie Allen, D.C. K. C. Chan, OMD., C.A., Jerry Green, Judy Gladstone, Dr. Raymond Castellino, Jo Ann Sorgman, director of the Santa Barbara College of Oriental Medicine, my devoted staff editors—for their strong support; and my former husband, Ted Bestani, whose love and expertise I could not have done without through this project.

The material contained in this manual has been researched, tested, and proven to be true in my personal experience, as well as in many offices, and has led to successful results. The key is not in the materials alone, but in how they are applied. In good faith, I share this information with you towards the purpose of opening your mind and heart to successfully doing what you most love to do in service.

—Cynthia Flint Bestani

Table of Contents

PERSONNEL--YOUR INVALUABLE SUPPORT

PRACTICE MANAGEMENT PERSPECTIVE

FREE SUPPLEMENT
Current Standard CPT Codes & Procedures

Introduction

The Practice Management Guide Series is about moving forward with ability and knowledge; intuition and vision; heart, integrity, and action! *Volume I* contains not only an awareness of what makes successful practice, but a format for planning and decision making so you can focus your energy effectively. Although the authors encourage you to use a highlighter pen and write in this book, a more extensive separate *Practice Management Plan Format* notebook with 22 divider sections has been created for use with *Volume I* if you chose.

This guide is designed for the full range of alternative health care practices—from small and very simple to the large multiple practitioner practice with its unique integrated systems. As you use this book, you will find the parts in this book which will stimulate new insight, direction, and procedures valuable for you. As your practice grows, the needs of your practice and procedures will change. You may find that management procedures mentioned or discussed in the book seemingly unnecessary now, will become vital as your practice grows. Many of these procedures provide the foundation and preparation to help you serve better and assist your practice to grow.

When you hire your office staff, I encourage you to let them handle the material presented in the manual series on office procedure operations and insurance. Keep freeing yourself up to handle the important decisions, and give yourself the gift of renewal. I also encourage you to take full advantage of the contents of this book. Test it out and expand it, and it will serve you well over many years.

I acknowledge you now for your willingness to fulfill your potential and serve in a much greater way.

--Cynthia Flint Bestani--

How To Start

AND

Successfully Manage

Your Practice

How to Catch the Essence of This Book!

A good time to read this material when you are fresh, receptive, and alert. It will give you a good lift into your day. In order to get perspective, deliberately set a time when you say "no" to everything else including interruptions, and create a specific time for yourself to "take stock and visualize your course of action. Working with this book is a catalyst for your practice. Think of it this way: 80% of what we do comes from the other 20%, which is formulating time. The quality of that 20% affects the success of the other 80% of your time. Taking the time to focus your attention on your plan of successful practice management procedure can set the way you carry out the other 80% of your practice time.

I believe in writing all over this book. Write notes in the margin. Use a yellow highlight pen. Underline. Fold back the tips of key pages. Circle passages, and particularly, fill in the blanks intended for your planning. Insert cards as markers, and attach tabs that stick up from the pages for instant references. An old Chinese proverb says, "The strongest memory is weaker than the palest ink." Use these tricks of the trade to emphasize to your mind what's important for continued use. Then use this book over and over again to energize and refocus your practice at all its stages.

You may feel anywhere from bold to cautious after working with this book. Keep the impetus. Yet remember: Try new ideas conservatively in terms of how they might be made to work in fact. Consider your plans with a mentor. You'll find out soon enough if your newly found plan is most workable for you. Enjoy your opportunities, advantages, and strengths as you increase your mastery in managing your professional practice.

. . . Then there is how to miss the essence of this book. . .

— Practitioner reads the book and doesn't recognize the professional application to his practice.
— Practitioner recognizes the importance of what he/she reads, but never thinks about it again.
— Practitioner makes notes for future reference but doesn't remember to refer to them.
— Practitioner resolves to apply the new knowledge but doesn't take the steps to carry it out.
— Practitioner takes steps to implement the new knowledge but, at the moment of actual use, decides to stay with the tried and familiar.

This is a new time in our lives, a time to let go what hasn't worked, add to what does work and enjoy it!

Throughout this book you will have an opportunity to look at your skills and abilities in depth. This book will give you a perspective on successful practice so that you may hone your skills and abilities. If you are working with the *Practice Management Plan Format* while reading this book, you will find your vision opening to new perspectives and will have an opportunity to be introspect, retrospect, and creative with your approach.

Everyone drawn to the health care field as a practitioner already has many skills and abilities. These skills abilities are refined and honed with experience and knowledge. Hopefully you will continue to grow in your passion for your profession, your desire to serve your fellow man, and open to ways which increase clear intention, inner and outer knowledge, as well as action.

The skills and abilities of a successful health care practitioner contain the following elements:

— A true desire to help people.

— A firm belief in the health care which you offer.

— Communication skills: the ability to have rapport, express oneself, and influence people.

— Knowledge and use of effective methods to change the patient 's attitude from symptoms, disease and medicine to cause, correction, health restoration, and health principles.

— He knows how to and does generate new patients without unethical advertising or gimmicks.

— He has a deep desire to be a consciously competent practitioner, who takes the time to meditate in his way, to be clear about his objectives and priorities, as well as balance and "tune" to the feeling tone and information around him. He is able to be in the flow with a sense of synchroncity and to integrate, communicate and act in a timely way and be in the flow.

— He learns to generate supportive teamwork and feedback to implement his practice plan and expand, grow and change with the needs of the time.

— He can keep a realistic overview. He is able to perceive the influencing intangible factors.

"HOW DO I FIT?"

Your Role

Whether you are a student considering your future, ready to start in practice or already in practice and considering new options, you are on an adventure which has a number of options. You will have an opportunity to explore which option will serve you either now or at an upcoming date. There will be most likely at least one option which can be to your best benefit. Your decision will most likely come down to one of these:

— To enjoy the security of working for another practitioner.

— To develop your techniques and business ability and model under another successful acupuncturist or health care provider.

— To practice on your own, if legal.

— To work in conjunction with an allied practitioner, perhaps in a shared space capacity, referral capacity, partnership, corporation, or buy-out situation.

The state or country in which you choose to receive your license will open up or limit your options. So laws and location will play a part in your decision, as well as personal desires, strengths and assets.

Now let's look at the possibilities. Read the section and then go back over it and ask yourself: "How did I react to the pluses and minuses?"

"Do I Want to Be In An Associate Program?"

First, we'll look at what an associate program is and how it works. An "Associate Program" is a program designed to strengthen and expand an office by qualified staff with different levels of function. The roles are intern, associate, colleague, and director. Built into the program are incentives such as further educational training, increased patient care, and advancement of position and salary. How does it work? We'll start with a few definitions based on a program which has a proven basis of success.

What If I become an Intern, Associate, or Colleague . . .?

4

Advantages

You...

1. Don't have to risk a large outlay of capital to make a practice work.

2. Don't have to have capital to sustain yourself through the first two years of the practice.

3. If the practice is down, it is more the director's responsibility to oversee and pick it up. As a colleague, you will want to take more responsibility, especially since your net is particularly affected.

4. Do what the director asks of you. You are more independent as a colleague.

5. Don't have the stress of ownership.

6. Make a net profit usually in your first week in practice, where as the owner may not in his or her first two years of practice.

7. Have a regular take home salary. As an associate you may have a percentage of the gross practice income or you may have a salary and a percentage. As a colleague you may receive 35% of net.

8. Don't have to be concerned with hiring, training or firing staff.

9. Have no money tied up in the practice. You don't have to buy equipment and meet mortgage payments.

10. May, as an associate, move into a colleague status usually within one year.

11. Have the education, mind, heart, and hands to heal, but do not have to have the responsibilities and directorship to handle public relations, financial affairs and running a business.

Disadvantages

You...

1. May want to control the way the practice is run and can't.

2. May not earn the money desired.

3. May not have control in the manner of treating the patients.

4. May not be able to utilize your full potential and may express frustration

5. May feel "unequal" and unmotivated to increase the patient volume if there is favoritism on the part of the front office staff towards the director or "other" staff over you.

6. May not have the challenges you want.

7. Cannot build a future private practice base from these patients. By virtue of a "No Competition Agreement," the patients belong to the current practice.

"Would I Want to Be a Director of An Associate Program?"

The considerations basically stem around the advantages and disadvantages of hiring associates. The main considerations in hiring an intern are : 1) They are there to provide basic support functions and 2) to learn to fit into how the office works.

They should not take on the managerial role of the office. That job should be given to a highly qualified manager. The considerations with colleagues usually will have worked out through the trial associate period. If you become a director, remember: Your staff is your backbone. If you provide them with good incentives, they will stay with you as a strong team.

Advantages of Hiring An Associate

1. It increases the director's practice and his/her income with little extra work and without patients dropping off.

2. The director makes a percentage of the associate practitioner's income as the associate increases his or her practice.

3.   The associate increases services to patients which also increases both associate and the director's income.

4.   The director can take vacations and have patients cared for while he or she is away, allowing for consistent patient care and an opportunity to relax and spend time with his or her family.

5.   It allows the director to handle an influx of new patients, and to treat patients who need more frequent care, without feeling overworked and exhausted.

6.   It allows the director the option to not turn away patients and enjoy the added professional assistance to treat more patients.

7.   It allows the facility to be used to maximum potential. The schedule can be opened up earlier in the AM, the lunch hour and the night hours can be covered, as well as the director's days off from the office.

8.   Space can be more efficiently used. Perhaps your current storage room can be better used as a treating room, and storage can be accommodated elsewhere in better used space.

9.   Staff can efficiently handle an associate; or perhaps additional staff can be easily added to accommodate an associate.

10.   Overhead at 55% warrants hiring an associate.

11.   Other conditions make it ripe such as: the dollar per case load averages is over $400 per case; the average visit is $40+; the average patient office visit is 15+ per patient; you have on average 30-35 new patients per month and can comfortably give 12-15 new patients to an associate. You have 120/140 patient visits per week in this scenario; you are willing to train an associate, and to risk losing a few patients in training an associate.

12.   If you, as the director, die, the practice would be valuable to an associate beyond the value of equipment and the office building. He/she could continue the practice on as before because of the element of good will established. An agreement could be worked out with the remaining spouse to buy the practice, thereby protecting the heir. If the associate had life insurance on the director, this would all pay for the cost of the practice in the event of death. The option, of course, would be selling to another unfamiliar practitioner

or reverting the equipment, etc. to the lender, if any. Passing the practice into the hands of the associate is far more preferable.

13. It keeps the director mentally stimulated with up to date information and practices. The director has the benefit of a second opinion on patient care.

14. It allows practitioners to specialize and practice what naturally is right for each one. Perhaps one provider specializes in female problems and child birth preparation, where another specializes in gastrointestinal disorders.

15. The associate is able to produce three times his salary if he is a good producer, thereby justifying his employment.

16. The director does not have to raise prices to an excessive level or work twice as hard to keep up with inflation or patient volume. In hiring an associate, the director's tax bracket may be more manageable too, because he/she can expand the practice without raising his/her tax bracket. The director can plan to level his/her income at a specific amount which would allow him/her to take home more and work less.

Disadvantages of Hiring An Associate

1. An associate may not be able to take directions.

2. The associate may not be a producer.

3. The director may not be increasing more patients consistently enough to warrant long term hiring of an associate.

4. An associate may not be motivated enough to generate the care of new patients.

5. Techniques or attitude may not be compatible enough with the original treating practitioner for the patients' satisfaction or the other practitioner's satisfaction.

6. The associate may leave prematurely.

7. The associate may develop divergent goals and cause conflict within the practice.

8. He or she may create insecurity in the director if the patients keep requesting to see the new associate rather than the director.

9. Resentment may be generated if the associate doesn't earn his dollar goals and there are no built in advantages to staying with the practice.

10. Staff conflict can be a major issue. The associate may terminate in the middle of training if he/she and the office manager or staff aren't in agreement on the way office policy and procedures are implemented.

"Should I Work With An Allied Practitioner?"
(MD., DC., DDS., Licenced Acupuncturist, etc.)

Various kinds of arrangements can be drawn up. Remember, the law in the state or country of your choice will influence what kind of arrangements you can make in your locale of choice. The options open to you may be:

1. An employee or contractor within the same office (colleague, associate, intern), whose patients belong to the clinic or director's practice.

2. A contractor within the same office, whose patient's are his own and do not in any way belong to the clinic or director's practice.

3. A solo practitioner who refers patients and is "referred to" within the same complex or at a location within the community.

4. A consultant or consultee.

    ★Note that the Contractor-Rental Agreement may be used to advantage between another practitioner and the acupuncturist if they are in the same office.

Advantages

Working in an office with an MD or other allied practitioners.

1. The MD. can provide valuable information on the patient's condition. (So can the other allied practitioners).

9

You, as an alternative or complementary practitioner:

2. Can have the added professional clout of being in an established practitioner's office, particularly if it is a successful, prospering practice.

3. Can have an understood referral base that is active.

4. Can have office use without owner overhead responsibilities.

5. Can use staff services such as some or most of the following: telephones answered, appointments made, bookkeeping services free or reduced health care for self and family.

6. Can receive a steady paycheck, i.e. every two weeks or as per contract if you are a colleague, associate, or intern.

Other advantages:

7. Insurance billing through a medical doctor.

8. The presence of a medical doctor in case of an emergency requiring other emergency support.

9. Building a patient practice quickly.

10. Advantages of colleague and associateships listed previously.

11. As an independent contractor within the same office , you have the advantage of your patients being your own, even though patients may be "shared." Unless otherwise agreed upon, this may remain so in the future.

Further advantages and disadvantages are listed under the heading: "Should I have an Office Away From Home?"

Why Would an Allied Practitioner Include You?

The same advantages and disadvantages of hiring an associate, colleague or independent contractor apply. Your qualifications may lgally allow you to perform duties that other allied practitioners may not be able to perform and visa versa. You may complement each other very well.

How to Negotiate Your Position in an Associate Program Or With Other Practitioners

In this section we have looked at the advantages and disadvantages of being part of an associate program. We have also looked at working with allied practitioners. There is a wise saying: "It's not what I have, it's what I have access to" that makes development and ease possible. This aplies in negotiating your position. If you choose to work with other practitioners either in your space or their space, ask yourself:

- What advantages are most important to me?
- How can this role best serve me?
- How can I best serve?
- What do I want?
- What must I have?
- What does the other party want?
- What must the other party have?
- What spirit of teamwork is present?

If you have decided to work with another practitioner, negotiate with the other party what would be a win-win situation. Go for what you want and never below what you must have. Otherwise, you will not be fulfilled, and ultimately no one wins. Build into your contract the opportunities and rewards of achieving what would meet the needs and desires of all parties concerned. Look at the contracts in the *Big Forms Packet.*[1] They may be what you want. Otherwise, use them as a base for designing a contract which works best for you. You may want to include in your contract some of the benefits in the Staff Policy in this volume. Remember, if you design your own contract to meet your needs, it can put you at an advantage. Just be sure that whatever contract you use, you consider having it previewed by a lawyer first.

Find the right situation for you. If your present situation or negotiations don't work for you, remember: There is one that will. Keep exploring your options and ask further questions. For example, "Am I best served by owning my practice?" We'll consider this next.

1 **Contracts:** Partnership Contract , Associate Contract, Colleague Contract, Independent Contractor Contract, No Competition Agreement. (Big Forms Packet From Tao to Earth, Focus PM Pubs. Distribution at 1 (800) 800-3139

Why Own Your Practice?

This section will give you a better idea of the benefits as well as the pitfalls involved in owning your practice. (There will be some variation in information according to your state or country regulations and changing law.)

Sole Proprietorship

Advantages

1. You are the boss. You have the control over what you financially put into your business, the management of your business, who you hire, and what responsibilities will be handled day to day.

2. You reap all the profits.

3. You personally know the employees and patients.

4. You can act quickly in decision making.

5. You are free from a lot of red tape.

6. You may pay less income tax than a corporation.

7. It's the easiest and quickest form of ownership to start. There are no contracts to draw up to start. Simply obtain your business licenses from your local or state offices, and you can begin.

Disadvantages

1. You may lack special skills and abilities. Perhaps you are excellent as a healer, but you lack the desire and knowhow as an employer, financial, operations, marketing, or public relations director/administrator.

2. You may lack funds, and the expansion may be slow.

3. You are at risk. You bear all losses.

4. Illness may close your business for a day, a week, a year, etc.

5. You are limited by your source of capital, your personal capital, earnings of the business, or the amount that can be borrowed.

6. A great deal of effort may yield little return particularly in the beginning. Your employees may reap greater financial reward than you as the employer, and you have all of the added responsibilites of a sole owner.

Partnerships

Advantages

1. You can pool your skills and abilities. You may be an excellent financial manager while your partner may be an excellent public relations person. Both of you may be excellent healers. You both can weigh the pros and cons in decision making with the business, as well as provide second opinions when treating patients.

2. Your combined sources of finances are increased.

3. Your credit position is improved for obtaining additional funds.

4. It magnifies the contribution of goodwill.

5. Partnership increases the concern for good business management.

6. It can be less of a tax burden than a corporation. Individual partners pay personal income tax on individual profits.

7. It is more flexible, less expensive and easier to modify than a corporation.

8. Competition may be eliminated when profits are shared.

9. One partner can retire, for example, from the management part of the business, but still be part of the business.

10. Partnership is beneficial to the operating economics. Group expenses, such as advertising costs, supplies, equipment, utilities, group furniture, and rent can be divided into group and individual expenses. A set amount can be provided in the budget for individual costs (education, periodicals etc.), and can be divided equally among partners.

*** Note the very general comparison to corporations and seek a lawyer or certified public accountant for more specific counsel.

Disadvantages

1.   Partnership can create unlimited financial liability for all debts. Each is responsible for his share; however, if one doesn't have the available capital, the others may have to pay all the debts and have a claim against the partner.

2.   There may be disagreements among partners. This could occur over the sharing of management responsibilities, over the kind of business practices, the direction of the business, the profits to share. This may be avoided by delineating specific duties of the partners.

3.   Each partner is bound by the contract of the others. If it relates to the operation of the business, there is the possibility of ill-will, if certain aspects of the contract turn out to be to the disadvantage of the other one or ones.

4.   Life is uncertain. If one dies, the heir may demand an unfair price or insist on ending the partnership. Insurance on each partner can be bought to cover the cost of the purchase price and should be done. Bankruptcy of one or an entrance of a bad partner may bring an end to the partnership when the business is doing very well.

5.   There may be an unsatisfactory division of profits. This may occur if one partner puts in more time and effort than the other or utilizes greater abilities than the other to reap larger profits.

6.   There may be difficulty in withdrawing one's share from the profits. There may be required approval by all of the partners.

7.   Even in a limited partnership, there is unlimited liability for debts unless there is a certificate of limited partnership filed in a public office of record and proper notice is given to each creditor with whom the limited partnership does business.

Corporations

The two main differences between these and other businesses are 1) the tax laws and 2) the law governing liability. Check with a lawyer or certified public accountant on these because the laws change as often as yearly.

Advantages

1. The source of capital can be increased by selling shares to stockholderers.

2. Owners (stockholders themselves) are not liable for debts of the corporation beyond the investment in stock. Your personal assets are protected.

3. One source states that the only reason to incorporate is to protect individuals from lawsuit and creditors and protect businesses which borrow a lot of risk capital.

4. Partners incorporate to protect the individual partners against certain types of lawsuits and losses from the action of the other partner or partners.

5. There is an ease in transferring ownership by selling the stock.

6. Permanency of existence. Death does not close the business or corporation, as may occur with sole proprietorships and partnerships.

7. Corporations are the only businesses that can hire employees, pay them a wage, and offer to them company paid fringe benefits such as health insurance. Every employee's wages, including the owners, are deductible as an expense to the business. Expenses reduce profits which mean lower income taxes to the corporation. (Wages are taxable to owner/employees as personal income). Certain fringe benefits paid to owners are tax deductible to the corporation and these fringe benefits are not taxable to the employee.

8. There are other specific tax advantages. Check with your attorney or certified public accountant for your specific situation.

Disadvantages

1. Although small corporations do have a few ways to reduce combined corporate and shareholders taxes, it may not result in taxes lower than those paid by unincorporated businesses. Consider this carefully.

2.   Incorporating does not protect you from malpractice suits.

3.   Although incorporating with the idea of protecting oneself with a large outlay of risk capital is a strong consideration, remember that the lender will require a guarantor of the loan and a financial commitment in case of change in ownership. You may be at risk more than you thought.

4.   Check with a corporate attorney or certified public accountant for your specific situation.

Subchapter S Corporations

Subchapter S Corporations have the same structure and similar benefits of a corporation. Subchapter S corporations do, however, have a maximum limit on the number of stockholders.

Advantages

1.   Subchapter S Corporations offer the same limited liability protection to stockholders as a corporation.

2.   Owners pay no corporate income taxes. Like a partnership, all profits go to the owners who are taxed at their regular individual rates.

3.   Distributions of profit are not double taxed as in a regular corporation.

4.   If there are no prior business tax years on which to carry back a loss, owners/stockholders can carry the loss back to their personal prior year returns, even though the business did not exist then.

Disadvantages

1.   Some states do not recognize Subchapter S Corporations and tax these businesses as regular corporations.

2.   Owner/employees of Subchapter S Corporations are not allowed all the fringe benefits available to owner/employees of regular corporations. Read the tax information on Sub S corporations in IRS Publication #589.

Should You Buy a Practice or Start from Scratch?

Buying a practice can have many advantages over starting from scratch if you have the money to borrow, pay cash, or invest. Number One: It's already set up for you. The question then becomes:

- Can I afford it?
- Where can I find one?
- Is it set up to my best advantage?
- Do I want to do it now, or position myself to work up to it?

Starting from scratch takes more effort, planning, set up consideration cost, building a patient base from zero, setting up new policies and procedures, equipment purchases and office staff. It may also be harder to get a loan for a new practice, than one already setup and thriving. However it's yours.

Advantages

1. You can profit from carrying forward and extending the former practitioner's goodwill and reputation of healing.

2. A good practitioner can build a strong referral base from the former practitioner's existing and recalled patients lists.

3. All of the equipment and staff may be readily available to use with little turn over needed.

4. The owner may be willing to finance at a lower rate than most lenders would, so it may be easier to buy a practice than start one from scratch financially.

5. If the practice is already profitable, this can be magnified further with little effort by refining treatment procedures, referral building, office efficiency, etc. and easily adding other practitioners.

6. It may have all the best features listed under "locating" your practice site, which would greatly enhance buying.

7. If the philosophy of the existing practitioner is consistent with yours, there is likely to be an easy transference from the former practitioner to you by his/her patients.

8. If the fee schedule is not too far off from what you would propose, this will assist in an easy transference.

9. If the financial policy is productively generating consistent revenue, this is to your advantage. See if the existing staff is carrying out good financial policy and if they are willing to adopt to changes you may make.

10. There is an equipment advantage if it is lien-free, in good repair, and useful to you.

11. There can be a tremendous overhead advantage assuming you can manage the outlay of capital. Notice: Are the utility bills reasonable? Are the lease agreements, if applicable, equitable? Does the insurance seem appropriate and in line with existing needs? Does overhead appear to be in line? Is the payroll acceptable to you?

12. A financial advantage is where the accounts receivable are three times the gross plus 10%.

13. Purchasing an office can have advantages in the appearance and layout you want to have, especially if it is already attractive or easily refurbished.

14. The cost advantage is when the practice is commensurate with its worth.

15. The owner may be willing to work with you on a 90 day transference, promoting you to the patients, allowing you to use his/her stationary, to deposit into your account checks which are made out to him/her on accounts receivable, etc.

16. The owner may be flexible on the purchase price, down payment, and other terms of buying the practice. He may respond favorably to negotiating with you equal tax advantages and disadvantages. (Note: Work with a C.P.A. on this, as well as a lawyer.)

17. An important advantage is where the owner signs a legally drawn up "no competition" agreement with a reasonable and legal mileage radius.

18. The owner also may be open to doing a gradual sale such as in the case of the owner retiring. This may also be an advantage.

Disadvantages

1. The practitioner may be selling a lemon.

2. Overhead may be too high.

3. The patient load may be low volume.

4. The practice may have a bad reputation.

5. The practice may have no reputation.

6. The location may be poor. There may be changing population in the neighborhood, rezoning, or reconstruction of a freeway through the site.

7. Industry may be waning.

8. The growth of the town may have leveled off.

9. The area may be too saturated with competition.

10. The bookkeeping system may be a mess. The accounts receivable may not be accurate. Many accounts may be old and non-collectible. If the practitioner has a poor reputation, you won't be able to collect on his/her debts.

11. There may be liens on the equipment.

12. The equipment may be in disrepair and require a large outlay to repair or replace.

13. His/her philosophy may be different and not compatible with yours, which would cause the patients to be unhappy.

14. Your practice management procedures may be tighter than the former practitioner's and cause ill feelings during the transition time and/or in the future.

15. You may be buying unnecessary equipment.

16. You may be buying too much stock, which has been or will sit unused, unproductive, and go bad.

17. You may be leasing unnecessary equipment.

18. The former expenditures may be way off from what you would spend. You may have to shift a lot of expenditures, sell old equipment and unused stock. The stock the owner valued may not have nearly the value to you.

19. You may have to rehire and train new staff if current staff isn't acceptable or workable for your needs.

20. The modalities may be different or nonexistent.

21. The fee schedule may be too different from yours.

22. Utility bills may be too high.

23. The accounts receivable, whether high or low, may prove to be high write-offs. Check on the ratio of collection to fees for services rendered, type of financial policy and agreements with patients, consistency and follow-through with payment plans and the aging of accounts status.

24. You may need to change the form of advertising if the cost outlay is too much with too little return.

25. This may be an acute care practice rather than a chronic patient practice, which means a high turnover in patients.

26. The office may need lots of upgrading, painting, and/or refurbishing.

27. Low accounts receivable may also indicate a high predominance of cash payers, out of balance with patients who could be attracted to continue needed care by establishing a third party pay system with some credit extension.

28. High accounts receivable could indicate poor collections, poor insurance billing practices, non-aged accounts, and old uncollectibles.

29. Patients may need too much retraining to be comfortable with your management practices of appointment scheduling, patient care program, or financial policies.

30. The practice selling price may be way off from what you would value the worth of the practice or even what a broker would value its worth.

These points were cited from Dr. Peter Fernandez, _How to Buy and Sell a Practice_, c. 1980. If you wish to pursue further buying or selling your practice, this book is excellent. It can be purchased from 7777 31st St. North, Suite 15, Seminole, FL 33776.

Are You A Candidate For Practice Ownership?

An entrepreneur --and that is what an owner becomes-- usually has a strong desire to be his own master. He typically can't be as happy working for others; He has a strong need for achievement; He is usually too creative to feel comfortable following out someone else's idea or procedures, and too decisive to wait for the slow wheels of an organization to turn before decision or changes can be made. An owner wants to make decisions, especially the kind of decisions that produce results at his own pace. He also wants to try out ideas and to have the freedom he could never have as an employee. Ownership often represents the fulfillment of a dream.

To be successful at owning your practice, ask yourself if you have or if you can easily develop the following abilities, resources, and assets which will lead you to success:

- Am I determined to learn, grow, and succeed in a practice?

- Do I possess self-knowledge, including acknowledging what I don't know?

- Am I consciously competent in my field and in regard to what creates health? do I have a good understanding of human behavior surrounding health, illness, and business issues?

- Am I good at overall planning and preparation?

- Am I a good at financial planning, funding, and financial management?

- Am I willing and interested enough to stay current with the changing needs and desires of the health care market and keep my skills updated?

- Do I exude a working smart, healthy, and happy philosophy?

- Do I have a good ability to listen for feedback and to make and act on decisions?

- Do I have a good ability to make myself understood, including my expectations and needs?

- Do I communicate effectively with a variety of people — not only patients, but employees, suppliers and lenders?

- Can I oversee, manage policies, set procedures, delegate them, and track the practice; or can I take the time to hire an excellent manager and others to do the things I am weak in or don't have time to do?

- Can I resolve my conflicts between business and personal goals?

- Can I handle an element of risk?

- Do I have a sense of my destiny--being in the right place, at the right time, doing the right thing for me?

Ownership starts with a desirable service, such as your health care services, and an effective marketing strategy for building both your reputation and a preference for your services. The successful owner must then prepare a detailed operating plan that includes types of services, treatment rationale, additional health product sales, policy and procedures, staffing, expenses and capital expenditures.

To achieve success a practice must be carefully planned and effectively managed. This will take important qualities such as perseverance, initiative, confidence, self-reliance, and the need to achieve, all of which are related to determination. Initially, an owner must assume responsibility for every detail of setup of policies, procedures, and operations, unless he/she has trained assistance. An owner must comply with a number of governmental regulations; obtain and maintain adequate financing and sources of supply and generate income and profit. He/she must be able to create enthusiastic patients, motivate staff, negotiate with vendors, and convince lenders. Aside from using his/her ability to inspire others and cope with the myriad of details and long hours at the beginning of practice, he knows that there is no guarantee of success. An owner-practitioner will see and at times experience that his services can decrease with unskilled or unmotivated front office management, poor communication, inadequate patient follow-through planning and care, referral building planning and follow-through, seasonal changes, or when the competition in the area offers better or more services, equipment, or more complete health care.

You can visualize, or at least glimpse, that an owner reaps all the joys, victories, benefits and rewards of ownership, but he also must contend with all the failures, limitations, and setbacks. He knows he can't be an expert in every business operation, and has to learn the delicate technique of delegating without abdicating. He must be able to bounce back, be able to suffer occasional defeats, perhaps even disasters, and still maintain his balance.

The successful owner is the one who is determined to learn from his or her problems and mistakes. He knows or comes to know his weaknesses, and makes sure he has effective backup partners, employees, or consultants. He listens to his patients, staff, and his accountant, and puts in the corrections to achieve success. He knows how important support is and how to appreciate those who are there for him. He generally has a strong support team with his family at the head of the list. He also seeks out or has other role models or a mentor whom he can turn to for advice.

Since management is the major reason for ownership success or failure, look at your determination to learn practice management and your willingness to follow-through to success in your current venture or in other ventures past. Is it strong?

Although the statistics for any given year are disheartening enough to discourage all but the hardiest from owning a practice, the good news for owners is that good management can be learned! With adequate awareness of some simple business principles, preparation, funding, good patient visit, referral, and treatment rationale, networking and outreach, checks and balances can be built into your practice for success! It takes you, as the practitioner-owner to listen to the feedback, and put in the "extras" which make your practice uniquely successful.

What to Get Legal Assistance On

When Setting Up Your Form of Business

Sole proprietorship seems like a fairly easy form of legal entity. However, there are many hidden factors to consider. For example, sole proprietorship does not always contain the best form of liability and risk protection nor does it always provide the greatest tax advantages. Because the legalities of starting in practice are so complex, we have composed a list of the considerations to work out with a professional legal adviser. Also included in this section are charts and articles appropriate to this section.

- ❏ Type of business entity appropriate for your needs
- ❏ Eligibility of owners and number of owners
- ❏ Classes of ownership interests
- ❏ "Flip-flop" of interests
- ❏ Liability of owners (limited liability, business debts, other)
- ❏ At risk rules (such as of Sec. 465)
- ❏ Rules for formation of the business entity you are considering
- ❏ Cost of formation of the business entity of choice
- ❏ Protection of your business name
- ❏ Restrictions and availability in raising investor capital
- ❏ Control of enterprise and investors
- ❏ Required and prohibited acts
- ❏ Participation in management
- ❏ How arbitration and settlement of disputes are handled
- ❏ Additions, alterations, modifications of agreements
- ❏ Ease and effect of transferability of interests and ownership
- ❏ Receipt of an option to acquire an interest in the entity as compensation for services
- ❏ Effect of death or sale of interest on basis of assets in business
- ❏ Rights of continuing partners
- ❏ How is sale of ownership and/or interest to take place, time limits
- ❏ Avoidance of liquidation (unlimited life and continuity)
- ❏ Revocation of pass-through status of continuing business
- ❏ Inadvertent termination of pass-through status
- ❏ Post termination transition period

- Income in year of death of an owner
- Cash distributions not changing relative interests
- Distribution of cash in redemption or decrease of interest in entity
- Adjustment to entity's basis in assets from outside events
- Owner basis as a limitation on losses; impact of entity debt
- Different distribution rights
- Distribution of earnings subsequent to year-end
- U.S. IRS or your country ruling policy on tax status
- Who pays what taxes
- Minimum tax on preferences
- Salaries paid to owners
- Earnings accumulation
- Passive investment income
- Selection of taxable year—restriction and non-restrictions
- Accounting methods and change in accounting methods of your existing business
- U.S. Federal, state income tax, and annual franchise tax. Other country: taxes
- Special allocation of items of income, deduction, and credit
- Specific dollar amount on certain deductions
- Charitable contributions
- Transfer of debt-encumbered assets to business
- Taxes on transfer of assets to business
- Tax-free reorganization
- Liquidation
- Distribution of appreciated property other than liquidation or tax-free reorganization
- Gain on sale of equity interest / loss on sale or worthlessness of equity interest
- Gain / loss on transactions between entity and owner
- Absence and disability arrangements among owners/employees
- Fringe benefits such as pension or profit-sharing plans, other
- Transfer for value rule of life insurance
- Social security taxes
- Reduction of social security benefits during ages 62-71

U.S. FORMATION OF A BUSINESS ENTITY

TYPES OF ENTITIES	SOLE PROPRIETORSHIP	GENERAL PARTNERSHIP	LIMITED PARTNERSHIP	CORPORATION
1. FORMATION	No formal steps except Fictitious Name Certificate	Usually written Agreement, can be oral	Written Agreement with Ltd. Partnership, Cert. recorded in counties where Partnership does business	Files Articles of Incorporation with Secretary of State
2. COST OF FORMATION	Nil	Costs of preparation of Agreements	Costs of preparation of Agreements	Filing fees plus legal fees
3. PROTECTION OF BUSINESS NAME	Fictitious Business Certificate	Fictitious Business Certificate	Fictitious Business Certificate	Articles of Incorporation
4. RESTRICTIONS IN RAISING INVESTOR CAPITAL	Depends	Depends	Depends	Yes
5. CONTROL OF ENTERPRISE/ INVESTORS	None	Agreement defines control	Limited Partners have very limited votes on Partnership matters	Shareholders have limited involvement in day to day business
6. BUSINESS DEBTS LIABILITIES	Yes	Yes	General Partner Yes; Limited Partner depends	Shareholders No
7. TRANSFER OF OWNERSHIP	Depends	Depends	Depends	Depends
8. TAX IMPACT	Owner	Owners	Owners	Corporation is the taxpayer
9. CONTINUITY OF LIFE	None	Depends	General Partner No; Limited Partner Yes	Yes
10. FRINGE BENEFITS	Retirement Plans	Same as Sole Proprietorship	Same as Sole Proprietorship	———

(SCORE REPRINT)

Note: There is some variation in different U.S. states.

How Necessary Is A
Written Partnership Agreement?

A written partnership agreement is always advisable. Business partnerships almost invariably begin with the highest of hopes and the best of intentions. The partners are thinking about business success; they don't want to even hear about disputes and buy-outs and dissolutions. That's understandable but it is not a businesslike approach to a serious business matter.

Look at it this way: Even if your business is successful (and there is no guarantee of that), few jointly owned businesses are owned by the original partners for more than a few years. A special opportunity may arise causing one of the partners to leave, a partner may grow tired of the enterprise or simply want out or, in those infrequent cases where a partnership endures unchanged, someone is going to have to deal with the eventual retirement or death of one of the partners.

All of these matters, which comprise the operation and termination of the partnership, should be spelled out in a written partnership agreement that is dated and signed by the parties involved. You may wish to consult an attorney to assist in the preparation of the agreement, but partners themselves can draft a suitable binding agreement that serves their respective interests and covers all major areas of concern.

Let's consider a few of the issues that should be addressed in your agreement:

" *Length of the partnership.* How long is the partnership to last? You may wish to be partners indefinitely, or you may wish to set a limited time period in the case of one partner who intends to leave.

" *Contributions of the partners.* What, specifically, will be the contributions of the partners to the enterprise? How much in the way of cash, property or services will be expected from each person? How much work will the partners be doing; will they be full-time or part time?

" *The need for more money.* If hard times threaten the future of the business, requiring an infusion of new funds, will the partners be required to contribute equally? What if one partner can't or won't?"

" *Distributing profits and losses.* How profits and losses are to be distributed must be decided. A closely related issue concerns salaries: are they to be paid to the partners, and if so, how much and on what basis?

" *Decision making.* How decisions are to be made must be stipulated. This can be handled by requiring unanimous agreement of the partners, but plenty of other methods are available. For example, you can designate decision-makers or you can provide for weighted votes depending on contributions to the partnership.

" *Disputes.* You must decide what will happen if there is a serious dispute between the partners. You can make no provision and therefore run the risk of costly litigation, or you can provide for binding arbitration or mediation as ways of resolving important disputes without the travail of a lawsuit.

" *Termination of the partnership.* What happens if one of the partners wants to quit, or dies? How is the value of the departing partner's interest to be determined? If the business breaks up, who owns the business name, the customer lists or other valuable assets?

These are painful issues to consider especially amid the euphoria that so often accompanies the start of a business. But think of it this way, a sound partnership agreement-one that carefully contemplates adversity-can be a key element in structuring long term business success. Keep in mind too that by mutual consent, partners can modify or rewrite their original agreement. The point is to create a written document that reflects a clear understanding of the rights and the responsibilities of the partners.

For further information, "The Partnership Book," by Denis Clifford and Ralph Warner (NOLO Press) is extremely helpful. It's available at your local bookstore.

By Larry Agran

Reprinted from the Los Angeles Times Home Magazine, June 20, 1982.

The Partnership

The Uniform Partnership Act, adopted by many states, defines a partnership as "an association of two or more persons to carry on as co-owners of a business for profit. "Though not specifically required by the Act, written Articles of Partnership are customarily executed. These articles outline the contribution by the partners into the business (whether financial, material or managerial) and generally delineate the roles of the partners in the business relationship. The following are example articles typically contained in a partnership agreement:

Name, Purpose, Domicile

Duration of Agreement

Character of Partners (general or limited, active or silent)

Contributions by Partners (at inception, at later date)

Business Expenses (how handled)

Authority (individual partner authority in conduct of business)

Separate Debts

Books, Records, and Method of Accounting

Division of Profits and Losses

Draws or Salaries

Rights of Continuing Partner

Death of a Partner (Dissolution and winding up)

Employee Management

Release of Debts

Sale of Partnership Interest

Arbitration

Additions, Alterations, Modifications of Partnership Agreement

Settlements of Disputes

Required and Prohibited Acts

Absence and Disability

Some of the characteristics that distinguish a partnership from other forms of business organization are the limited life of a partnership, unlimited liability of at least one partner, co-ownership of the assets, mutual agency, share of management, and share in partnership profits.

Kinds of Partners:

Ostensible Partner. Active and known as a partner.

Active Partner. May or may not be ostensible as well.

Secret Partner. Active but not known or held out as a partner.

Dormant Partner. Inactive and not known or held out as a partner.

Silent Partner. Inactive (but may be known to be a partner.

Nominal Partner (Partner by Estoppel). Not a true partner in any sense, not being a party to the partnership agreement. However, a nominal partner holds himself or herself out as a partner, or permits others to make such representation by the use of his/her name or otherwise. Therefore, a nominal partner is liable as if he or she were a partner to third persons who have given credit to the actual or supposed truth of such representation.

Subpartner. One who, not being a member of the part-nership, contracts with one of the partners in reference to participation in the interest of such partner in the firm's business and profits.

Limited or Special Partner. Assuming compliance with the statutory formalities, the limited partner risks only his or her agreed investment in the business. As long as he or she does not participate in the management and control of the enterprise or in the conduct of its business, the limited partner is generally not subject to the same liabilities as a general partner.

From the pamphlet on "Legal Structures of Business" by the Small Business Administration

PLANNING YOUR PRACTICE

Planning for Different Stages of Practice

While you are in school, considerable amount of planning should be done before even thinking about setting up a practice. Part of clinic lends itself well to preparation, especially to patient treatment and care. However, so often the pressures of studies crowd out the other types of planning that should be done early on, and a number of practitioners rush into practice as soon as they get their licenses. Many who finally open their practice aren't aware that successful practices plan in specific phases both before and after opening practice. They are stumped with the predicament in which they find themselves. The problem with the lack of awareness of planning for practice stages is that practice management becomes "crisis management." It becomes mostly a relief care type of practice, while not ever getting to the cause of successful practice.

Decisions, policies and procedures which work best at one stage of practice must give way to those which work better at another stage. To plan most effectively, shifts in planning must be made at each stage to prepare to move into the next stage.

At each stage carefully look at what you want to do, the future impacts, and how you will achieve what you want with your practice. How does it fit with your personal and other professional goals? This may determine how committed you are to doing what you say you want to do. Identify: 1) your strengths and weak areas, 2) how you can best use your strengths, 3) how you can find complements for your weak areas, and finally 4) how you can receive the support you need for moving into the next practice stage.

What Are the Stages of Practice?

For our purposes here, we'll call the practice stages:

- Pre-start up: early, middle, final initial planning stages.
- Opening practice to cash flow stabilization stage.
- Stabilization.
- Stabilization to growth.
- Plateau.
- Growth to expansion.
- Expansion to leveling off.

Pre-Start Up: Early, Middle, and Final Initial Planning Stages

Often in the early stages there is an inspired sense of direction. You move into a course of study, trusting that it will lead to fulfillment in some way and prove to be a good occupation. Once upon the course of study, it can have an all-consuming effect, depending on the rigor of the program. However, take the time to look carefully at how the scope of practice you undertake can best be used. Focusing on "specialties" within the study can be used to unique advantage. This may take a little research. As a result, you may even decide to take additional or complementary classes to give you additional expertise before you open your practice. Begin to consider what equipment and health care products can best support the way you want to practice.

Through training in the area of patient management, you will be setting up standards and procedures for patient care, and feeling the kind of rapport you want to have with patients. Your treatment rationale will formulate. This will include: 1) the type of recommendations you will make 2) the plan you will use to recommend beyond relief care, 3) your plan to promote follow-through, and 4) you will choose the forms to use for patient care which you will adjust to suit your purposes. You will learn about front office procedure in school. *The Front Office Procedure* text is useful.

The early stages is the time to take advantage of observing other clinics to see front office procedure and flow in motion, and to see how other practitioners carry out their treatment rationale and build loyal referrers.

The early planning stage is the time to carefully consider where you will get your license so your location fits the way you want to practice.

View it from the standpoint of the legal scope of practice, not just emotional preference. Scope out the success of practices in the location of your choice and begin researching the qualities of potential patients in the location you will eventually practice.

In the middle planning stage you will be exploring various roles. Important questions to consider are: "Is it in the highest interest for me to work in an associateship program? Should I start a practice in my own space? Should I share space ? Is it more feasible to start from scratch or buy a practice? Is it to best advantage to do this alone, in partnership, or as a corporation?" If you choose to practice in an associateship program, you will look to see with whom you will practice, what you will do, and where you will go to find your practice of choice. You can then negotiate your position.

If you choose to practice on your own, you will first be looking at the money available to start a practice, where and how to borrow funds, and how to pay the money back in a timely way. Pencil in the figures to see how much money must be put aside to sustain a practice in the period in which it takes to build stable cash flow and give you a good salary. It could take 6 to 18 months to stabilize.

The middle planning stage for those who want to practice on their own involves research phone calls and getting very specific data for a marketing and financial plan. It is recommended to do 1) demographic and psychographic data of your potential patients in the location of your choice. 2) a survey of the competition, complimentary practitioners, and success of other like practices in the area and 3) a survey of the fee base in the area. This is the time to set up your niche for the location and get clear on your unique advantage. (This is well described under the marketing, location, and fee headings of this book.)

It's time to get as realistic a picture as possible about financial costs. Pencil in specific financial costs for equipment purchasing, office set up costs, health care products outlay, and the cost of renting or leasing different types of offices. Ask:

> What can be added and what should be trimmed to 1) give the greatest service 2) easiest financial flow and return at the start of practice and then at the stabilization stage of practice?"

Get clear on your objectives and goals in each area of practice so that you will be able to start putting together your plan. (See "Creating a Practice" and planning sections at the end of various chapters to include with the outline plan.)

Assess the financial impact of your plan, and get ready to submit your plan for funding. Research possible office arrangements and scope out potential rental arrangements.

Before financial, location, and practitioner arrangements are set, all plans and contracts should be reviewed by a professional financial planner, SCORE free service agency representative, accountant and a lawyer for potential flaws.

In the later pre-start up phase, funding arrangements are made; contracts are signed; and equipment, office supplies, bookkeeping systems, and patient forms are purchased.

This is the time you want to ask for help and spend time fixing up your potential space, and setting your equipment and supplies in place. You will be setting the atmosphere and image you want to convey. If you are renting in another office part-time, you may not have much freedom to shift items in the treatment room. However, it can be done.

In the beginning you may not have a front office staff unless you are sharing staff. Get feedback on how to organize your office/treatment space to work to best advantage. How do you want front office procedure to enhance the vision of your practice? If you share front office staff with another practitioner, it's to your advantage to spend some time educating the staff to your needs. It's worth it in order to receive the quality of communication and rapport you will need.

Spend worthwhile time and energy educating your assistant about your 1) objectives, 2) needs, and 3) goals. This is an important time of establishing policy, procedure, and the tone and image you want your practice to convey.

You can best use the **Volume II** to advantage at this point with your assistant. If you don't have an assistant at this stage, do the review in **Volume II** for your own clarity. Review how safe practice works; protocol for office flow, how practice building occurs with telephone procedure; time slotting for patients; how follow-through is promoted in scheduling, how financial policies, fees, and collections will be handled, how patient orientation, education, and referral building procedure will take place, how paperwork will be processed; how insurance will be handled; how to promote stabilization of income; control inventory, and keep on top of the bookkeeping. If and when you have staff, address the importance of keeping practice management control records and giving you feedback in regular meetings. Provide a staff policy and show your staff how he/ she will benefit from your practice growth. Plan what your staff needs to know to promote good patient intake, phone, scheduling, collections, and patient follow-through procedure with care. This is the time to put financial management and appointment management control forms in place so your staff can track your income and other statistics.

Initial Start Up

Much of the policy, procedure set up, and planning is done. The initial stage is the time for a practitioner and his assistant to: 1) set up speaking and demonstration engagements for you, 2) arrange meetings with those in your referral base, 3) and study and refine procedures. Promotional materials to reach your potential patient can be added and refined.

In the beginning you may spend more time networking out of the office than in the office. This is the time to influence. Visit other clinics, educate them about what you do, offer a class, and build your referral base. Your promotional efforts will gradually take hold and patients will begin to schedule.

This is the time to set your treatment rationale and approach in motion with good patient rapport, health care planning, report of findings, directions, recommendations, multiple treatment scheduling, communication with concurrent practitioners, etc.

To move toward stability, build a practice from your strong areas and complement by referring out in areas you are not competent or equipped to handle. Focus on quality service and successful results with patients. Build a history of success and begin creating a good reputation.

I f you have staff, meet with them on a regular basis to hone and refine the rough areas of the practice. Improve telephone, scheduling, and patient care procedures.

Gear financial policies to stabilize cash flow and promote towards specialties which ensure cash flow. If you haven't learned the art of referral, learn how to build patient rapport and how to educate your patients to refer. Your patients are the ones who will build 75% of your practice. Your own referral building detector must be awake and alert to build your practice. The types of patients which you have and build in the beginning will set the tone for future referrals.

Stabilization

As the practice builds, it will reach a point of financial stability. Treatment procedure and service quality is honed to be consistently good and reliable. Efficiency and effectiveness are part of the practice by the point of stabilization. You succeed at this stage by looking at your appointment book and tracking stats over time. Notice the patterns of stabilization. Redirect your energy as needed. When the practice income and expenses have stabilized, you can begin to liberalize your financial policy and extend credit in other forms. You begin to "plan growth."

Stabilization to Growth

This is the stage of "planned" growth. As procedures are refined, more is accomplished in less time. Planned growth means gradually adding staff hours to accommodate growth with quality care and perhaps a part-time insurance clerk to handle greater insurance processing. This is the time to preserve quality, safe practice, and your reputation.

Pay close attention during this time to "follow-through care," particularly as the practice gets busier. Omissions with your patients can make your practice drop. Call backs must still be timely, cancellations rescheduled, "backsliding prevention" maintained. Avoid over booking. Expand practice hours or cluster patients to accommodate peak times. Rely on group health care classes for patient orientation, education, and invitations to friends and family. Use audiovisual aids to further educate your patients.

The primary office assistant should be good enough at this point to take on greater responsibilities of management. Building teamwork and increased communication is important during this time, particularly as this is a time of quickening pace and change. Staff development and greater teamwork is required for referral building to occur. Referral building is specifically geared towards the specialties of choice. Keep up on collections, and follow-up on insurance as the practice gets busier. Growth must not cause financial management to lag. Maintain accurate recording, even if this means adding more staff hours. Continual daily feedback from staff and patients is vital during this period.

Plateau

Practices slow down particularly when there is poor referral-building procedure or *no* referral-building procedure. Practices they also slow down with specific seasonal slumps if there has been no planning for seasonal changes. Practices also reach a plateau when the extras which were part of the practice in the beginning begin to slide or when boredom sets in. If staff has been overworked, they will often slow the practice down by the nature of their rapport and scheduling.

A plateau cycle can be an indication that it's time to take stock of the practice and assess what works best with the practice and what works least. It can be a time to consider weeding out dead end procedures, consider the best use of roles, hours, workdays, and assess one's promotion and approach, etc. It's more a time of consideration. Outwardly it's not particularly an active time.

Plateaus are often inwardly a creative time of contemplation, assessment, and a time to let a new cycle emerge. Take a short time off during this stage, perhaps have another practitioner fill in for you. Coming out of a plateau cycle usually occurs when one begins to integrate changes one at a time. It can also take the form of great resurgence.

Resurgence into Growth or New Areas

Developing a new interest in another specialty, fixing up the office, rearranging the furniture, changing an old image which doesn't fit any-more, or simply updating the practice is enough for the practice to take a new turn. Often when a practitioner takes a seminar, his practice will spurn onward again with renewed interest. New thinking even about standard methods can revitalize a practice.

Front office staff and other professional staff will usually recharge with a staff picnic, special luncheon, meetings outside the office, birthday celebrations, and when given a focus of related educational videos, audios, management books or seminars related to their office or practice experience. Professional seminars, collection seminars, practice management seminars and staff meetings keep the fire cooking.

An urgency may occur to create a legacy or make a profound difference, and at this stage, you may move into growth again with the decision to expand. For some the turn may be to do research part time.

With others, there's a focus on a new specialty area of practice. It could be writing part-time regarding their discoveries or experience and/or teaching about it. A number of practitioners will still maintain their home base practice part-time and open an additional practice in another area. Some decide to sell their practice and move into a completely new area of experience.

Expansion

The expansion cycle begins when you find it's time to add new practitioners to your practice. Professional staff training and development is emphasized, and the model which was set in the first few cycles is readied for associates and colleagues to participate. Expansion may further occur if a particular model warrants expanding into offices in other areas. An owner acupuncturist will move more into the role of director and provide more of a coordinating or teaching role.

Expansion to Leveling Off

Often a practitioner who has been in the field 15 years has more of a sense of completion. At this stage you may consider selling your practice, cut way down on practicing, and spend more time doing what you had initiated in an earlier cycle such as writing, teaching and doing other things with your life.

What stage of practice are you? _____
_____

What are your immediate goals? _____
_____
_____

How will you expand to the next stage? _____
_____
_____
_____

> *If you are at the pre-start up phase, the next section of the book will be particularly applicable to you. Otherwise, turn to the sections in the book which are of greatest interest to you at your stage of practice.*

Use this section as a checkoff list for starting in practice.

❑ 1. Get an understanding of the basis of successful practice. We'll be looking at these in the upcoming sections.

❑ 2. Decide what role you will perform:
   A. I will/ will not be practicing as ❑ an independent contractor ❑ with/without another practitioner; ❑ an employee in an ❑ intern   ❑ associate   ❑ colleague capacity.
   B Interview acupuncturists or other health care practitioners to see with whom you fit.

   C. Review the business relationship contracts in the *Big Forms Packet.*

❑ 3. Decide what business form you will practicer: I will/ will not be practicing as a ❑ sole proprietor ❑ partner or as ❑ an acupuncture corporation.

❑ 4. Determine where you want to practice. It may be most advantageous to pass your examination and obtain licensure in the state you would   like to practice.
   ❑ a. What is your location: _____
   ❑ b. What are your specialties and form of practice presentation?
   ❑ c. Survey and identify your advantage in relation to demographics and psychographics of your potential patient.
   ❑ d. Survey and identify your advantage in relation to the com petition.
   ❑ e. I plan to ❑ use a home-office combination ❑ lease ❑ rent ❑ buy a building
   ❑ f. I plan / do not plan to ❑ buy a practice
   ❑ g. Use the criteria on location and office space, to get clear on the site.

❑ 5. Create your practice plan.
   Purchase an 81/2" X 11" Notebook at least 3 " thick and title it: "(Name)_____'s Personal Practice Notebook". Set up index tabs in the book for each of the headings listed in the format of the "Practice Plan Outline". Buy pocket folders to put under the different sections, and insert into the

pockets relevant material specific for that heading. Creating the notebook will assist you in making the material in the guide "yours", as well as help you focus on an area one at a time.

Fill in your business plan whether you are starting your own practice or participating in your acupuncturist-employer's business plan. You will be more part of the practice if you are aware of various aspects of how it works. Even if you are not now an owner of the practice, learn as much as you can about it. You may at some point want to be a partner in your acupuncturist-employer's practice or start your own practice.

❑ 6. Use a "Weekly Plan" and "To Do List " to accomplish your objectives.(Copies in *Volume II*).

❑ 7. Identify your resources and develop your rapport with the following:
   ❑ The Acupuncturist's Practice Management Guide Series.
   ❑ College or continuing education instructor of health care practice management
   ❑ Free community services which offer assistance to small businesses
   ❑ Practice management services
   ❑ Loan officer or banker
   ❑ Accountant or bookkeeper
   ❑ Lawyer
   ❑ Business consultant or financial planner
   ❑ Marketing advisor
   ❑ In-house staff

If there is a continuing education practice management class at your nearest acupuncture college, take the course. Discussing and visualizing the material will assist you to make it real for you. The support in beginning your practice can not be underestimated. Talk with other successful acupuncturists, and ask them what works for them in their practices. They were once starting out as you are, and remember the pangs of starting a practice. They may be willing to share their experiences with you. If you feel uncomfortable with this or look upon this as an intrusion, attend meetings where successful acupuncturists speak on beginning their practices.

❑ 8. Use the Format for "Income and Expense Planning," including the practice income wheel and estimates of expenses.

❑ 9. Survey the fees in the area. Set your fees and financial policies. Post your professional fee schedule and financial policies where you and your staff can use them. (Note format for setting fees and financial policies in this volume.)

❑ 10. Research where and how to get your funding, and fill out necessary paperwork for a practice loan.

❑ 11. Assess your office space needs. Research potential spaces if you plan to rent, lease, or buy a space or a practice. (Use checklists in *Vol. I*).

❑ 12. Check into sources and costs for insurances you need, as well as business licenses. Make the necessary arrangements after review.

❑ 13. Make sure your financial plan is reviewed by a professional business advisor. Do this after you have filled out your practice plan and determined the amount of funding with which you think you have to work. Make sure all legal contracts are reviewed with a lawyer and though through carefully before they are signed. These are ownership, employer-employee contracts, rent/lease or purchase contracts, loan contracts.

❑ 14. After you are clear on your overall budget, purchase your equipment your bookkeeping system, supplies, and business forms . Allow enough time to get your printing done regrading checks, appointment cards, and forms before you open your practice.

❑ 15. Consider how your patient record forms will best serve you now. (When you have staff, train them how and why to use them.

❑ 16. Prepare ahead for a clear treatment program. Set up your treatment and health care planning system, scheduling system. Use the "18 safe practice communication guidelines" and forms (*Vol I & IV, Big Forms Packet)*.

❑ 17. Consider carefully what your professional identity and image is. Develop a marketing plan, patient education, and a referral program utilizing (Use Volume I tools and especially *Volume IV, Patient Communication, Public Relations, and Marketing*)

❑ 18. Set your practice hours and the way you want to function time-wise in your practice.

❑ 19. Have your brochure and other educational and promotional pamphlets and advertising reviewed first by someone knowledgeable in the field; then print your materials. Advertise when you are ready to open.

❑ 20. Be familiar with how front office procedures work for new and established patients, who do and do not have insurance. If this is not your forte, hire or share front office staff who are well trained. He/she should be trained in appointment scheduling and phone procedure, the way your financial policies work; how to use your fee schedule, bookkeeping system, fee slips; handle collections and billing; know how to relate with insurance companies and insurance billing procedures, organize your office, and do practice management control procedures; use safe guidelines which prevent malpractice; and know how to build referrals, assist in patient education, and keep your office running smoothly. (Volume II The Acupuncturist's Front Office Procedure Manual is excellent training for you and/or your staff.)

❑ 21. Use the safe practice guideline, particularly in staff training.

❑ 22. Start building your referral base with practitioners and contacts.

❑ 23. Understand along with your staff the way insurance works. *Volume III The Acupuncturist's Success with Insurance Guide* go into the specifics.

❑ 24. Use the staff meeting guidelines in this volume and meet regularly to train and develop your staff's abilities and ensure good communication and team spirit.

❑ 25. Set up your practice management control forms and get feedback. Monitor your practice.

❑ 26. <u>Give excellent patient care.</u> Notice what patient care procedures in "What Makes Practices Grow" and in the procedures section of "Income Planning" add value to your practice.

Why Create a Practice Plan? What makes it Successful?

Most practitioners want to be healers first, handle operations second, and do practice administration and management last. Can this work? With insightful thinking and planning, you can arrange your time, energy and resources so that you are devoting most of it to your first love while still running a successful practice.

Every practitioner is able to visualize the practice in which he can benefit others and fulfill some part of himself. This visualization is important because it is this ideal scene that reinforces our purpose when the short term frustrations and failures arise. They key to success after visualization is insightful thinking, strategic planning; exposing yourself to the conditions of the marketplace; and selecting the best way to carry forward your purpose, objectives and goals. Your practice plan is a vehicle for this process.

In the beginning of practice you have more time to investigate alternatives and set the major course of your practice. A practice plan can help you anticipate the important decisions you must make and help you give these decisions the proper attention they deserve.

Insight thinking is thinking which discovers opportunities, advantages and strengths and uses them to turn resources into assets which will provide stability, planned growth, and expansion. Insight thinking selects resources which inspire and create:

1. Cooperation.
2. Successful results.   5. Patient and staff loyalty and enthusiasm.
3. Reputation.   6. Referrals, and in turn,
4. Follow-through care   7. A Profit.

A practitioner uses insight thinking to weigh the type of available resources. He does strategic planning to set a number of intangible and tangible assets in place, which he monitors and adjusts as needed. Using insight thinking and strategic planning with these seven criteria in mind creates successful practice plans and successful practice.

Creating a practice business plan will expose you to where and what your health care market is like, financing requirements, personal considerations, profits, and problems. It stimulates what you can expect in the early months and years of operations. It "grounds" your planning. A well-formulated plan prepares you for the expected and frees your energy to handle the unexpected.

A practice business plan includes your objectives, goals, and financial projections. It is the framework which you make up which can tell you and others:

1. What conditions are ripe for your venture.
2. Where you will locate.
3. How your scope of practice will fit in.
4. What services you will offer.
5. What your marketing, advertising, and funding plans are.
6. What your business projections of expenses and income are.
7. What your fee structure, your policies, and procedures will be.
8. Whom you will delegate what aspects of your business to assist you.
9. What management controls you will use to monitor your business.

This plan can communicate the believability of a successful business proposition to your lenders. When you present your plan, it can show them:

1. You are confident enough to lead.
2. Rational enough to realistically plan.
3. Orderly enough to present your plan properly.
4. Your plan can provide a base for credit extension from your suppliers.
5. It can be used as a communication tool to orient personnel regarding your intentions, objects, and goals.

Your business plan gives you practice in thinking about conducive and competitive conditions, and when necessary, it gives you information to change the course you initiated. Your practice management plan scan help you make business decisions more objectively, rather than from strictly intuitive emotional feelings. It can provide a focus so you can renegotiate the use of your time and resources to fulfill your purpose, carry intention into action, and achieve your goals. Your management feedback controls will also show you where your obstacles are so you can put in the corrections.

Best of all, by using your practice plan, you will be able to look back at what you set out to do and appreciate all you have accomplished. This is remarkable with all its ups and downs, discomforts and rewards. For it's the victories of the human spirit that make a practice what it is--throughout all its stages. They are victories from planning and negotiating to creating and designing your space; from achieving success with patients to building your reputation. They are your victories from acting in clarity, learning humility in ignorance, expressing compassionate in your humanness. They are your victories in inspiring to others and expanding your work and gratitude in prosperity--an of your work and your prosperity -- An ordinary man taking opportunities of greatness.

Outline for Your Practice Plan

The information in this book will provide you with the necessary information, forms and tools to put together a practice plan outlined below. This is the format you also include with a loan package to financially fund your practice. Practice plans vary in length and nature.

1. **Resume**
    Personal Name. Address. Phone. Date. Personal Data. Education. Professional Experience. Licenses. Memberships. Post graduate courses. Avocations.

2. **Professional Statement**
    Your purpose, objectives, and goals.

3. **The Profession**
    Background. Current status of acupuncture; state openness to acupuncture and the scope of the law there as it relates to acupuncture; trends in the medical field and how acupuncture fits; future prospects of services and response. What will affect these.

4. **Scope of Your Practice**
    Include a statement of your practice brochure on how you treat, the equipment you use, and how your training applies.

5. **Projected Treatment Rationale**
    Type of health care planning you will emphasize---%relief; stabilization; optimal care; maintenance care; preventive care. Will you do examination such as by level of complexity and diagnosis; treatment rationale? Will you do report of finds, home care recommendations and products, give directions, do multiple appointment scheduling; reevaluation of progress?

6. **Your Services and Health Products**
    Acupuncture services and other modalities you will bill. Health products you will sell. Include volume, number of new patients per month, expected income from examination, treatments, modalities, health care products. Inventory costs and risks.

7. **Market Research and Analysis**
    Data on the locale and potential need of the location and people for your

services. (Information from the Department of Health and Chamber of Commerce on demographic and psychographic data, health problems, health needs, population analysis).

Competition; market size in potential patients and dollars; demographic and psychographics of potential marketing niche. State the source of your data--Health Department, government reports, acupuncture associations, health care magazines, other magazines, reports. Include projected market growth in 3-5 years by what you have read.

8. **Marketing Plan**
    Your approach; methods you will use; advertising; promotion; service policies.

9. **Financial Plan**
    Include the financial impact of demographic and psychographic study of potential patient and location. Services, procedures, policies, location, office presentation and image, marketing.

    Long range and short range goal planning and costs. Cash flow analysis (Patient type, volume, turnover rate, marketing and referral building procedure for new patient development. Financial policy. Balance of accounts receivable to cash. Cash to expenses.)

    Break-even and profit analysis.
    (See financial management section. Note management control forms).

10. **Proposed Financing of the Practice**
    Desired financing. Use of funds.

11. **Management Team**
    Key job of staff. Management responsibilities. Hours.

12. **Supporting Professional Assistance**
    Accountant, lawyer, banker, insurance agent; business assistance services, consultant.

13. **Location Plan**
    Geographical location. Why this geographical and office locale. Office location: pictures of your office, drawings of your office size and layout, number of rooms, type of complex, leasehold improvements

type of lease and signs. Facilities and improvements planned. Operations strategy: lease, rent, buy, future considerations.

14 . **Equipment, Furnishings, Supplies Requirements:**
Reception area furnishings. Examination / treatment / dressing room equipment and supplies. Business furnishings, equipment, and small supplies. Professional resource materials. Therapy equipment. Consultation room furnishings and miscellaneous items. Miscellaneous and inventory of health care products.

15. **Professional Fee Schedule**

16. **Financial Bookkeeping System and Policies**
See office policy brochure in *Big Forms Packet or Volume II.*

17. **Patient Orientation and Education**
Health care classes; pamphlets; videos.

18. **Insurance Program**
Type, policy, and promotion.

19. **Service and Products Development**
What you will increase and decrease with stabilization, growth, and expansion.

20. **How you will Monitor Practice**
Such as: management control forms, patient questionnaire, staff meetings, personal/staff and patient feedback.

21. **Legal Structure of the Practice**
Sole proprietorship; partnership; sub-S corporation, etc.

22. **Business Projections:**
Projected first year expenses. Projected initial opening, monthly practice, personal expenses. Special events.

The areas you will be developing:
1. Your vision for your practice: your services, your staff, time and resources.
2. Patient orientation and patient management.
3. Image, reputation, and a successful position in the market.
4. Your income and expense set up and management.
5. The ability to build and monitor your practice.

RESOURCES

Using Your Greatest Resources
to Create Successful Practice

Your Unique Advantage Type
Type of services, specialties and health care products which make you unique, easily defined, and which match the demographics and psychographics of the patient market and location.

Impacts: filling a community need; practice financial stability, growth, and expansion; type of patients and referrals; ability to generate volume, and hence, revenue and cash flow; professional fulfillment.

Communication and image   (positive, neutral, negative)
Affects degree of credibility, trust and rapport, type of patient attraction, perceived value by patient, fee base; impacts turnover, patient returns, referrals, volume, possible collection problems if staff or patients are disquieted.

Practitioner's Attitude
Affects perception of self, others and practice; ability to affect successful patient care, satisfaction, loyalty, enthusiasm; impacts development of referral base and life long referring relationships; affects type and quality of practice; determines ease and clarity of procedures and rapport impacts cooperation, patient type, turnover, type of volume, cash flow, cash balance, crisis vs. planned stabilization, growth, and expansion, and leveling off.

Staff Attitude, Presentation, and Rapport   (See Volume II)
Impact: Patient satisfaction, enthusiasm, loyalty, follow-through with care, referrals, minimal collection problems.

How You Reinforce your Image and Build your Reputation
Can strongly increase visibility, credibility, feeling tone of patient's experience positively, neutrally, negatively; can increase referrals, type of patients attracted, justify fee base and income level; influence type of turnover, chronic/acute care balance, response.

Patient Management Program
Increases services, reputation, quality of relationship, added value, justifies fees; loyalty of patient base, income by diagnostic program, acute care/chronic care balance impacts success rate, referral rate, type of patients referred and attracted, steady volume, turnover rate, increase and stability of income level.

Right Personnel, Generating Services and Income

Impact: Image, reputation, and revenues; not only saves error, lost revenue, prevents patient omissions, builds in good reputation, revenues, growth and expansion.

Building a Loyal Patient Program of Referral

High results, low cost. Effective, caring communication—steady referrals—growth with good reputation and prosperity.

Careful Advertising & Marketing Contact

Conscientiousness of high ethical standards with non-excessive action is important. Impacts: can increase visibility, credibility, accessibility, break down barrier of unknown reputation, can increase new patient volume, income.

Keeping the Larger Perspective of Practice Management

Influence: crisis vs. planned stabilization, growth, and expansion; sets direction and emphasis of practice and procedures; determines type of teamwork, clarity and ease of procedures, and quality control of the practice; affects ability to input timely adjustments and corrections.

Role

Impacts: personal satisfaction and professional fulfillment, degree of risk or incentive for financial or overall practice development, current level and future prospects for income growth, tax planning and advantages.

Location

Accelerated access by patient/area preferences for your specialty or services, can increase visibility, accessibility, credibility, image. Justifies fee base.

Office Appearance, Furnishings, Image Building Design

Impacts: image and type of patient attracted; builds in limitation or growth potential regarding who you want to attract.

Office Contracts (buying, renting, leasing, staff contract, renters and subletters)

Impacts: level of financial pressure you are willing to handle to stabilize, grow, or expand your practice. Immediate and future cash flow from professionals who rent from you. Possible tax advantages.

Considerations: long term financial and other commitments, functionality of office, capacity problems; return of steady income from office investment; ability to grow and expand skills or income from associateship program or renters. Impacts pace of financial risk and income. Has tax implications.

Equipment

Must be leased or purchased wisely to not offset inflow and outflow of cash balance; must monitor if it increases patient volume and/or income to justify choice of purchase or leasing. Equipment impacts: better service and income. Income from equipment use should be higher than lease payment.

Patient Orientation & Education Program

Increases reputation, quality service, educated referrals, volume.

Effective Telephone Set-Up

Determines reachability, image of availability in time of patient need, privacy, confidentiality. Best use for maximizing incoming calls and contact, ease of outgoing calls for collections, insurance calls, and problem solving. Reduces problems requiring phone communication; impacts: patient confidence and security. Speed of handling emergencies, malpractice prevention, increased patient volume. Reduces aggravation and delays in patient scheduling, in collection of payments, and contributes to patient flow and cash flow.

Effective Telephone Procedure (See Volume II)

High result, low cost. Impacts: new and established patient trust, enthusiasm and loyalty, patient volume, referrals, and reputation, and in turn increased income.

Appointment Management Program (See Volume II)

Impact: sets pace in the practice. Can increase good follow-through care, value, steady volume.

Accurate and Accountable Patient Records System (See Volume II)

Impacts: office efficiency and impression of accountability. Prevents potential legal problems regarding payment by insurance company or court.

Clearly Defined Type of Financial System

Impacts cash flow stabilization and ability to grow and expand

■ Cash practice only	High % collections, good cash flow least growth potential
■ Easy credit practice	High growth potential, greatest accounts receivable and bad debts
■ Sliding fee basis	Unstable income, tends to create welfare practice
■ Modified credit practice is the best balance of the first two above	

Fee Base (Regular, incentive and reduced fee services)
Impact: increases incentives for higher cashflow. Fees for services can impact patient's comfort zone in follow-through care.

Clearly Defined & Broad Financial Payment Options
Increases accounts receivable, permits follow-through care, and financial manageability for the patient.

Specific Financial Policy and Promotion
Emphasize according to practice stage. Policy impacts: cash flow, accounts receivable amount, financial options to start or continue treatment. Promotion impacts: volume of new patients.

Liberalized Defined Insurance Policy
Accelerate as good cash flow stabilization permits. Impacts patient financial management and financial ease of follow-through care; increases practice accounts receivable. High financial yield with billing efficiency and staff accuracy, communications, and follow-through.

Efficient Bookkeeping System
Impacts: prevention of lost revenue. Accountability; timely ability to keep the practice on track financially.

Use of Clear, Complete Written Service Charges by Practitioner
Efficiency, recaptured income – recovers potential lost revenue; increases swiftness of payment from patients or companies. Impact: positive cash flow, accurate recording – evidence of specific value given to the patient, effectiveness.

Consistency in Billing, Collections and Follow-through Procedure on Accounts Receivables (See Volume II)
High financial yield, low cost. Impact: increases cash flow; minimizes collection delay and problems.

Financial Management
Impact: ability to achieve financial stabilization, growth, and expansion.

The Essentials for Practice Growth and Profitability

Practices grow because of good patient care, the quality of service, reputation, image, the type of market addressed, the "preferred" specialty emphasized, the type of health care planning adopted, and the way referral building, marketing, and advertising are used. In each section of the book we will address how this occurs.

The attitude of both the practitioner and the staff are key. Positive outlook draws people to you. As you see people as a one of a kind unique human being, and not a case, they will feel it. As you sincerely want to learn what people need, why they need it, when they need it, and how you can help them achieve it, your natural communication about how this can occur can open the doors for this patient, for their enthusiasm, their loyalty, and in turn their referrals. As you keep patient care in balance with practice management, your practice can grow successfully in goodwill, reputation, referrals, and profitability.

When you study throughout this volume what can be done to increase practice growth, you will be able to include many new ideas and procedures as they are natural to you. These will succeed as they pass the tests of producing cooperation, results, reputation; and increase follow-through care, lifelong relationship, and referrals. Whatever you do to grow, inspire health, clarity, ease, and love of life.

There will always be the patients who switch, telephone shoppers who are just fishing, no shows, and procrastinators, do-it yourselfers, and deadbeats no matter what you do. Don't let these behaviors dominate your thinking. Growth isn't a matter of doing the "perfect thing" and being accepted and approved of by patients all the time. Focus on appreciation for those who do respond, and give your best.

Be assured that the major factors which create successful practice and practice growth also create profitable practice. *However,* practice growth does not necessarily equal profit. This is why growth must be planned. The following areas will be addressed to assist you to understand, create, and build a practice which both grows and profits. These are:

■ Managing cash flow proportion
■ Selection of income generating factors

- Expense control
- Ability to create a preference for your services and health care products
- Quality control of services, orientation, education, and care
- Steady referral base

For practices to grow and profit, it will be valuable to keep statistics. Simple statistics are a way to monitor your growth and guide your practice in a way that is more manageable. There's no need to get caught in the management control forms and try to manipulate numbers of patients or dollar signs because of what you find. You may however, need to make adjustments for cash flow stability and to keep up the quality of care. Practices grow primarily because of the attitude of *care* the acupuncturist and staff have when they do what they do. Management control forms can be most valuable if they motivate, reinforce, and shift *attitudes* which influence more effective results in the practice.

Concentration of Energy and Resources

A wise practitioner establishes habit patterns, thinking patterns, and practice patterns carefully and early in his practice. He works simply and concentrates his efforts. He takes time to consider what he must learn, arrange, and guide. How is this most effectively achieved? In the *Time Trap,* Alex Mackenzie points out a principle called the Pareto principle: 20% of a person's time present in concentration, envisioning, and planning will determine the way the other 80% of his time, and his staff's, is carries out. This is focused intent with processional effect.

He treats his time and his staff's time as valuable to fulfillment of purpose and enjoys what he does. His form of time management develops from the art and ability to concentrate–from no-mind to mindfulness. To achieve his best results, he generally orders his practice plan when he is fresh, rested and inspired. His actions spring from clarity, not from rambling from event to event.

Wise practitioners take the time to investigate and consider the right use of services, procedures, products. They consider those which bring forth the criteria of success we have spoken of – cooperation, reputation, results, follow-through care, life long relations, referral, as well as income. Those procedures are highest priority. If procedures do not meet this test, they are weeded out or not employed. They assess demographics and psychographics to set their location, office space, and fees. Then they are prepared to put effective marketing methods in place. They check financial costs, overview them, and wisely invest in capital and small expenses in a way that does not harm cash flow. They set financial policies to stabilize cash flow. They expand the accounts receivables at the rate the practice can extend credit. They take the time to build in safe practice procedures and appropriate time slotting of patients.

Wise practitioners build in financial and appointment management control forms, and take time to review them and make adjustments. They see: "To go wrong and not to alter one's course can definitely be defined going wrong. Those who will not see and do not act are as much a fool." [1]

They value well trained and developed staff who promote resoluteness, loyalty and enthusiasm, and in turn, follow-through and referrals. They plan time to better their staff and staff's performance. They plan patient orientation, health care programs, education, and referral building into their practices.

---

1 *Kung Fu Meditations,* Ellen Kei Hua, editor

They ask questions and provide their own answers to:

> What do I want to experience?
> What is most important now?
> What could I leave out now?
> What would create less hassle now?
> What would create greater fulfillment?
> Does this fit with my practice objectives and goals?
> Does this meet my criteria for practice success?

Successful practitioners get to the office early so they can move clearly into their day. They consider their daily schedule so they do not scatter their energy. They often use a daily and monthly calendar book for planning their personal and professional life. They manage their time in clusters of activities. They keep the practice on track by scheduling practice management review. They schedule regular meetings with staff. Their priorities are to heal, to achieve their goals, and fulfill their objectives. They are tuned to keep the practice on course and communicate to inspire the best in others.

Supporting Your Professional Goals

Most people, let alone practitioners, are normally strong in some areas and weaker in others. To effectively use time, money and energy, people can be your greatest allies. There are three main ways this is accomplished:

■ 1. Hire outside professionals to fill your needs on an hourly or piece basis.
■ 2. Hire in-house personnel, full or part-time.
■ 3. Handle it yourself or within your family.

Since there isn't time to do all things, and some of your weaker areas are better handled by others who are more competent in an area, you must delegate those areas to which you either shouldn't devote your energy or else don't prefer to devote your time. It is vital, if you are to turn your resources and potential liabilities into assets, to hire people who are competent in the area you want to fill. Pay scale should be according to the level of expertise required. If you hire weak people in areas you are weak in or don't have time to handle, you may find yourself calling in a consultant to get you out of the mess. If you try to handle it all yourself, or within your family, you may find yourself really not saving, time, energy, and money in the end.

The key in good practice management is to delegate according to competency level. Hire high competency staff and professionals in areas which affect profitability and growth.

Consider your ability to serve within the practice. For example, if you hire an ad agency on a percentage basis, to help you put together effective advertising which causes an influx of new patients, you must be ready to handle this within your practice.

Since patient rapport, telephone promotion, referral building and follow-through scheduling, affect your practice growth dramatically, hire a competent in house front office person from the stabilization to the growth and expansion stage. (Before you hire and delegate, be sure to read the section on hiring and delegating in the volume.)

Your Practice Team

These are the names of who you are or will be working with:

☐ Free services like SCORE —Service Corp of Retired Executives who offer community services to assist new businesses_____

☐ Loan officer or banker:_____

☐ An accountant:_____

☐ A lawyer_____

☐ Marketing advisor _____

☐ Insurance agent _____

☐ Practice management services for your specific profession:
_____

☐ Staff --full time _____

☐ Staff --part time _____
_____
_____

Where to Find Your Financial Resources

The following ways can be used to obtain money for opening or expanding your practice.

1. **Savings Passbook Loans.**
   You can borrow up to the amount you have saved -- even if your credit is bad. This is usually a quick bank loan with one day processing by your bank.

2. **Charge Cards.**
   (Mastercard, Visa). Obtain these if you don't have them. They establish your credit, and you can draw cash advances up to the maximum if necessary. You can have several cards from different banks and borrow against each of them. You can usually have your limit raised every six months upon request. Just be aware that the interest rate you pay on these are usually higher than other means of borrowing.

3. **Automatic Overdrafts.**
   You can apply for automatic overdrafts usually after you have received a check guarantee card and Mastercard or Visa from the bank. Then you can write checks greater than the balance in your account with limits that vary up to about $15,000. This is instant cash for you and no credit checking is involved once you are approved for automatic overdrafts. The bank may assign a limit which can be raised, if that is their policy.

4. **Travel and Entertainment Cards.**
   (American Express, Diner's Club, Carte Blanche). These allow advances often to $2,500. The Gold American Express card may go up to $5,000. This is instantly available money once you have obtained the card. (These may have to be paid off in full when you receive your bill, however.)

5. **Revolving Charge accounts.**
   (Sears, Montgomery Wards). These can be used to finance office supplies and furnishings.

6. **Cash Value of Life Insurance Policies.**
   These are fairly easy to obtain and at low rates of interest.

7. **Collateral Loan.**
   You can borrow against valuable jewelry, your automobile, heirlooms, paintings, household furnishings.

8. **Mortgage and Second Mortgages.**
   If your home or land is not mortgaged, you could mortgage it. If it is, you can take a second mortgage on it, or consider what you paid as well as the appreciation gained over the years and refinance the house or land for a larger amount. Check to see if interest rates are down now and what the trend is.

9. **Financing or Leaseback of Assets.**
   (Financial Firms, Leasing Companies). Financing or leasing is often a better way to go than outright buying equipment when you start in practice because it keeps your initial cost down. Which way is the best one in your individual case should be discussed with your CPA. The I.R.S. Code Sec. 168 and 179 allows an accelerated write-off which can make financing favorable over leasing. Under the new tax law, write-off's are even greater when financing.

   The positives for leaseback are that you don't have any of your money tied up on your equipment and you can lease for a longer time period than a bank will. The negative is that the interest rate can be almost double the bank's rate so you are paying an inflated cost for your equipment.

   After you have considered whether leaseback or financing is better for you, check with all your equipment suppliers for names of I companies who will either finance or sell and lease back equipment to you. Check with five or six finance companies at least to see if they will help you get started. You will need to qualify for either approach. One may be easier to qualify than the other. You'll have the see what the requirements of different companies are. Your fixed assets can be turned into quick cash.

   You must provide these companies with a list of assets, original prices paid and documented correctly. The leasing company will provide you with a contract for the sale of the assets and another contract describing the terms of the leaseback. The agreement can also make provision for you to purchase the assets for a specific sum when the lease period is over.

Check to make sure what you sign is workable for you. Does it work in considering your tax structure? Are your accountant and lawyer informed before you sign anything? Once you sign the paperwork, a check from the leasing or finance company is available to you.

10. **Trade Services and Credit.**
Trade carpentry, remodeling services, advertising services, bookkeeping, interior decorating services, janitorial services — all for health services.

11. **Accounts Receivables as Collateral.**
If you are a practitioner in practice or about to buy a practice, try using the receivables as collateral for a bank loan.

12. **Refinancing existing loans.**
If you have already been given a loan and have proven to be a good credit risk, it is not difficult to refinance your loan, either by the same bank or a different bank. Find out how much the paperwork costs and if there is a penalty for refinancing a loan before going ahead and doing it. Sometimes you can come out ahead refinancing a loan because it may be at a lower interest rate at a time frame that works for you.

13. **Commercial Bank Loan.**
Although many of the 15,000 commercial banks in the U.S. loan against adequate security, many will make character loans to a good risk. With an excellent credit rating and presentation to your loan officer, you stand a good chance of getting a loan. Loan officers consider practitioners to be a good personal credit risk. A local loan officer can often help you obtain a quick personal, uncollateralized loan for $25,000. If you have used charge accounts in the last few years and paid all your bills promptly, your area credit bureau will rate you higher than normal. When you inquire about bank loans, find out in what kind of loans that particular bank specializes. Some banks specialize in small loans. Others specialize in strictly million dollar loans, or auto loans. Don't give up. Talk to every bank in your community until you find the one who will give you a good starter loan. Make sure, if you get a loan, that you come with 1) your overall expense projections, 2) equipment lists, and 3) from where and from whom you intend to purchase your supplies. Some banks will lend you money at a reasonable buy-back and over a long period of time.

14. **Small Business Administration Loan.**
Call the Chamber of Commerce in your area regarding where the

Small Business Administration is in your area. These loans can be applied for directly through the government or through a commercial bank. These loans can take anywhere from two to six months to obtain and are limited in number and budget beginning with their fiscal year, so apply well in advance of starting your practice.

15. Relatives.

About fifty percent of practitioners get partial financing from their families. Families can be a great help in borrowing money. Ask if any of your relatives will co-sign a loan for you, loan you funds outright, or offer you a gift in assisting you to get started.

16. Partnership Loan.

This could be an active partner or a silent partner. There are investors who specialize in providing capital for sound ventures and a well organized practice qualifies as a sound investment to many. The loan could be over a term (say two years) or on demand basis (with a specific number of days notice) as circumstances dictate. If your partner or investor is another practitioner like yourself, make sure you draw up a contract and have it checked by a lawyer.

17. Government Assistance.

Check into the many government assistance plans available. Check with SCORE (The Service Corp of Retired Executives), the Small Business Administration, and the Department of Employment.

18. Purchase Money Mortgage.

If you are buying a practice, the seller may want to carry the mortgage himself. You may be able to buy a practice with a good interest rate over a long period of time, pay him/her monthly. This would avoid having to obtain a bank loan or going through intensive credit rating checks.

19. Negotiating Office Space Contract

Ask your potential landlord or landlady if he or she would reduce the rate of the office space lease payments for the first six months of your practice and increase it by the reduced amount the following six months on a two years lease. It has even happened that landlords or landladies have allowed the first six months rent-free until the practitioner got started: This may be a tax advantage to the landlord. If you can create value for the landlord as well as yourself, you can negotiate an arrangement that works.

These 19 sources have been cited from Dr. Fernandez, "How To Start A Profitable Practice From Scratch".

ASSETS AND LIABILITIES

Practice Insurance

Many practitioner associations are making business insurance available to their members, offering the best coverage. Check with your local and National Acupuncture Associations for availability. Otherwise, local insurance agencies offer combined business insurance policies.

Liability Insurance
Regardless of owning, renting or leasing an office, an acupuncturist should have public liability insurance on the office building and grounds, (his/her) automobile, liability resulting from the acupuncturist or (his/her) assistant's personal activities not related directly to the profession, or any accident occurring on the grounds in which neglect can be proved—property damage, including your equipment, or personal injury.

Automobile Liability
Any employee who uses an acupuncturist's vehicle in performing services for the acupuncturist should be coinsured in the acupuncturist's policy. The acupuncturist could be sued as well as the employee if an accident occurs. Also, the acupuncturist should consider coverage while driving a borrowed or rented auto.

Fire, Theft, and Vandalism Insurance
This includes such things as your building, furniture, equipment, all records and files and other contents of the office. Your accounts receivable files should be amply protected with a fire proof ledger box. Your file storage cabinet should be fireproof casing. Ask before you buy it. Those insurance companies which cover you generally will offer a comprehensive policy that includes the above liability protections at a premium far less than for separate policies.

Workers' Compensation Insurance
Most states require workers' compensation coverage on any employee working in a practitioner's office. Make sure that you and your spouse, as owners of the business, are covered. This is not always automatically covered. Research this. It's worth the investment of time and money.

Employee Protection Insurance
Protection and fringe benefits included here for the employee are life insurance, major medical insurance, disability insurance, and hospitaliza-

tion insurances. Often these insurances offered through a practice will be the only insurance your employee has.

Business Overhead Insurance
For this insurance you must be able to verify your monthly overhead expenses such as rent, salaries, utilities and other fixed expenses. This insurance covers loss from sickness or accident where overhead expenses continue even though the acupuncturist has no income.

Fidelity Bonds
This covers any employee who may prove to be dishonest. This is simply just good business practice.

Personal and Family Insurance
This includes family automobile insurance, fire and theft, public liability insurance and varying home owner related insurances, accident and health, disability, life insurance and major medical insurance for the acupuncturist and family.

Professional Liability Malpractice Insurance
Malpractice insurance is essential. It covers the acupuncturist for any mistakes that he makes on a patient, or any imagined mistakes on the part of a patient. This could be an accident, or an act of negligence by the acupuncturist, an associate, or assistant employed by the acupuncturist. It could be caused because of accident , resulting when some form of therapy or treatment is used or performed incorrectly, or an unsterile instrument results in infection.

Pay your premiums on time and keep even older policies on file. Claims may be presented years after either a real or imagined incident is filed.

Each state has its own statue of limitations on malpractice claims. The time limit for filing varies. Check with your state. If the injured party is a minor, the statute of limitations usually does not start until the minor becomes of legal age.

Keep thorough and accurate notes. This is one of your best protections. Under malpractice insurance, additional coverage may be purchased to protect you against assault, slander or libel. Often your professional association will have the best coverage on malpractice insurance.

Paraphrased material is from "Insurance" and "Malpractice Considerations", _Chiropractic Parapro-fessional Manual, Practice Administration and Management,_ used by permission of the publisher, the American Chiropractic Association, with author's responsibility for edited material, c. 1978

Tax Planning to Do

Who should deal with business taxes?
You, management or other professional help. Plan and delegate!

What taxes?
For the business itself, labor and other taxes these include:

- For the business itself:
  1. Sole proprietorship   - Form 1040/540
  2. Partnership   - Form 1065/565
  3. Corporation   - Form 1120/100
  4. Corporation Sub S   - Form 1120S/100

- For labor: payroll for employees and independent contractors

- Other: Sales tax, personal property tax, business taxes and licenses and self-employment social security tax.

Why pay taxes ?
There is a requirement of our system for voluntary reporting and periodic audits and for imposing penalties for non-reporting and misrepresentation. Ignorance of tax requirements is not acceptable. The person and business benefits of paying taxes are that 1) It is evidence of how you are doing. 2) Your filled in tax forms can assist you with creditors and obtaining credit.

When do you pay taxes?
Before the fact, not after. It's faster! Pay as you go and estimate taxes due. Plan opportunities to minimize taxes.

How to pay taxes?
Intelligently! Take it one step at a time. Plan and delegate the bookkeeping, and have a certified public accountant finalize tax reporting. Use your elections wisely. Your elections are: the cash vs. accrual, valuation of inventory, depreciation methods, and year end elections. Utilize your legal advantages, such as credits and retirement plans.

How To Prepare For Taxes

1. Use a budget so you keep your expenses in line with real income. Keep realistic income and expense projections. Balance necessary preparation and expansion of your practice. In the process, you must think in terms of real dollars. For every dollar you receive, you have X per cent of fixed expenses with X amount of variable expenses. Remember, taxes and inflation need to be accounted from every dollar you receive.

2. Seek the advice of a good tax accountant and financial planner so that you will be on top of it for tax preparation. You can't afford not to!

3. Hire a bookkeeper. Many practices have a competent family member do the bookkeeping. An acupuncturist has too many duties to hold onto the job of bookkeeping. The time is better spent on practicing and promoting your practice. You must, however, oversee the bookkeeping. Having your bookkeeping kept up to date will make tax paying easier for you.

4. Educate yourself on the basic tax deductions so you and your bookkeeper know what to record on your bookkeeping system. There are a number of excellent layman's guide books out on the subject. These can be purchased through your local book store. The Internal Revenue Service also distributes pamphlets which explain tax deductions and credits. These can be obtained free of charge from the IRS.

   If you'd rather not deal with tax issues and problems, make sure your bookkeeper, who records your figures, is well-educated in this and keeps you on track.

5. Regarding employee taxes: Let a knowledgeable bookkeeper handle this as well. Just make sure the taxes and tax forms are submitted on time or you will be penalized by the government.

6. Most accounting sheets are designed so that your bookkeeper can plug the figures directly into the tax forms. However, tax law has become more and more complex, so it may be wisest to give your quarterly and yearly figures to your tax preparer and have him or her do this for you.

7. Your past years tax forms will be useful in establishing credit. You will usually need to supply the last two years of tax forms to apply for a loan.

Employer and Employee Taxes

Have your office manager handle these details of payroll if (he/she) is versed in doing payroll. If you don't feel comfortable with this and you don't want to deal with it, there are companies which do this for you, i.e. Employee Management Corporation. They are here to uncomplicate your business.

Employee Taxes: (Also see the section of "How to Handle Payroll".)
Form W-4 or W-4A
Remember to have all new employees complete and sign a form W-4 or W-4A when they start work.   You should have a form W-4 or W-4A, Employee's Withholding Allowance Certificate, on file for each employee. Forms W-4 and 4A claiming exemption from withholding must be renewed annually. Copies of Forms W-4 or 4A received during the quarter that claim 11 or more withholding allowances must be submitted to the Internal Revenue Service.   In addition, copies of Forms W-4 or W-4A must be submitted to the Internal Revenue Service for employees who claim exempt from withholding and who usually earn more than $200 per week.

Federal Withholding and FICA
Obtain your federal withholding FICA pamphlets (Circular E) from your local IRS office. The amount of tax liability determines the frequency of deposits.   You owe these taxes when you pay the wages (date of check), not when your payroll period ends. Payments of federal taxes must be deposited with an authorized commercial depository (i.e., your bank). A federal tax deposit coupon must accompany each deposit.   There is a penalty on any deposit not received directly by the IRS, unless you have a reasonable cause. Check your federal withholding pamphlets yearly to determine when you do not need to deposit taxes, at what dollar amount you do, and how it is set up.

Federal Unemployment (FUTA) and State Unemployment Tax
Federal unemployment taxes are paid by the employer on a specific portion of each employee's annual wages. Generally there is a state unemployment tax in addition to the federal unemployment tax on the employees annual wages. Check federal and state payroll guides regarding current rates and taxable wage base, and how to handle payment deposits.

State Withholding Tax, State Disability Insurance, and Workers' Compensation Insurance

Check with a local state tax office, Labor Board, or certified public accountant to determine if you are required to have these coverages. Federal income tax withholding tables, Circular E, are revised yearly and state income tax withholding tables may be also. Be sure to use the table that is current as of the date of the payroll check. These can be obtained from your IRS and state tax offices.

Business Tax Deductions

Accounting fees
Advertising and promotional fees
Amortization of leasehold improvements
Bad debts from sales or services
Bank service charges
Bookkeeping
Books
Car and truck expenses
Casualty and theft Losses
Commissions
Computer services
Contributions
Depletion
Depreciation of property (i.e. buildings, autos, furniture and equipment)
Dues and publications
Education (for advancement and specialization) expenses / transportation
Employee Benefit Programs
Employment agency fees
Employee business expenses (reimbursed)
Freight
Flowers, gifts, and gratuities
Insurance
Interest on business loans
Janitorial services

Laundry and cleaning
Legal and professional services
License fees
Mortgage interest
Moving expenses i.e. equipment,
Night protection services (night watchman, burglar alarms, or guard dog services)
Office equipment rental
Office expenses - stationary, etc.
Office-in-home expenses
Office refurbishing
Pension and profit-sharing plans for employees
Printing
Rent on business property
Repairs
Research, development and experimental costs
Safe deposit box for items producing taxable income
Supplies
Taxes
Travel and Entertainment expense
Wages for employees
Work clothes-uniforms

Tax Deductions for Retirement and Other Benefit Plans

If you are self-employed, which includes being an owner or a partner of an unincorporated business, you may provide for your retirement by setting up either a Keogh plan or an individual retirement plan. Under the Self-Employed Individuals Tax Retirement Act of 1962, you are allowed to put a portion of your yearly earned income, on a tax deferred basis, into a fund that can earn tax-free income until it starts paying out of retirement.

You are eligible up to age 70 1/2 for an individual retirement account (IRA). An IRA is deductible as an adjustment on your 1040 tax form. There are some limitations on the amount that can be adjusted.

Under both an IRA and a Keogh plan, a portion of your income is sheltered from current taxation; there is no tax on the earnings of the fund until post retirement distribution (with the exception regarding early withdrawal); and qualified contributions made by employers to provide employees with retirement benefits are deductible by the employer up to specific amounts. Both Keogh plans and IRAs allow the self-employed owner of a business to shelter current earned income and allow that income to accumulate and earn currently nontaxable income until post retirement distribution.

The primary difference between a Keogh plan and an IRA is the amount of earnings that may be sheltered and the amount allowable as a tax deduction for the year. See your tax adviser regarding what would be appropriate for you. Another difference between IRA and Keogh plans is that if you are an employer, you may set up an individual retirement account for yourself without setting up a similar one for your employees. With a Keogh plan you must cover your employees.

It is almost always financially superior to adopt either an individual retirement account or a Keogh plan rather than have no plan at all. An exception would be a case when the after-tax cash remaining from funds not invested in an IRA or Keogh plan could be invested in a project whose yield would exceed, after taxes, both the amount that could be earned on the qualified retirement investment and the amount initially lost in taxes. For additional information on Individual Retirement Arrangement Deductions (IRAs, including the Simplified Employee Pension plan), see IRS Publication 590. For more details on deductions for Self-Employed Retirement Plans such as Keogh defined contribution plans and defined benefit plans, see the IRS Publication 560.

Aside from the tax benefits of retirement plans, an employer may also benefit from tax breaks for employer paid uniform allowances, health plans and group term life insurance which cover employees. According to the type of business setup, employers may be covered on some of these plans and derive better tax deductions, i.e. for medical insurance, on the IRS Schedule C than Schedule A medical deductions. See your financial planner/tax adviser to assist you in how to set up these arrangements.

Tax Deduction for Business Use of the Home or Rental

If you use a portion of your home regularly and exclusively for business purposes, you may deduct a pro rata portion of the operating expenses attributable to your home. The qualifying allocatable business expenses are deductible only if the portion of your home is used regularly and exclusively as 1) your principal place of business, and 2) a place of business that is used by your patients, clients, or customers in meeting and dealing with you in the normal course of your business, or 3) a structure separated from the rest of your living quarters. (i.e., It should be a separate room or at least marked off by a room divider or screen on a regular and exclusive basis and is for the convenience of the employer under a written agreement requiring this arrangement). The problem of proving how much room is used for business purposes can be overcome by the use of photographs.

You cannot deduct a portion of a dwelling unit where it is used for both personal and business purposes (i.e., a den or bedroom). You may deduct the storage space you use as a portion of your house to store products that are sold for resale or wholesale.

Included in the tax deduction is the proportionate share of utilities, water and sewer charges, repairs, carpet cleaning, etc., that is allocated to the office space. In all cases, the maximum deduction for the business use of a taxpayer's home may not exceed the amount of gross income less real estate taxes and mortgage interest. See IRS Tax Publication 587.

Who will you have assist you with tax planning? _____

_____

What State and Local Licenses You Need

Where to Obtain Your State Licenses.
You can call information to get the address of the particular state licensing committee you need. Applicant Instructions for licensure can be obtained from the Medical Board or appropriate governing body within each individual state.

Strictly Observe Federal Regulations.
The federal Food and Drug Administration regulations for herbs, acupuncture devices and importation of acupuncture supplies can be obtained by writing to the F.D.A. in Washington, D.C.

Obtain Your Local Business Tax and Permit Licensing.

1. **Business licenses.**
   Anyone conducting a business of any kind in the city is required to obtain a business permit and to pay an annual business tax. The taxpayer is required to submit a business tax application to the business tax office. Professionals such as acupuncturists pay a flat fee annually. If you are in an unincorporated county, requirements may vary. Check with your county or the appropriate government office for your state.

2. **Partnership and fictitious name business registration**
   You must register and pay a fee to the county or a state department, such as the Department of Commerce and Consumer Affairs. A fictitious name, i.e., DBA (Doing Business As), might simply be a store name or a combination or abbreviation of two partner names. Check with your county or state for their required procedures for registration and payment.

3. **Zoning requirements.**
   Contact the city or county zoning department to make certain that your business location is zoned for your practice and for the type of building and parking arrangement that you want to use.

4. **Building permits.**
   Any work, such as structural work to your office involving a change of use or occupancy in any building or portion of a structure inside the

city limits, requires a building permit from an office equivalent to the Division of Land Use Controls or in your city. Information as to whether the proposed use constitutes a change can be obtained by contacting the above. This department may also regulate signs. For county permits, approval is usually first necessary from the Planning and Zoning Department; following, a building permit will be issued by the Building Department.

5. **Health permits.**

Contact your government health department to determine if a health permit is required. Familiarize yourself with your state's Occupational Safety Health Act, which sets down exact requirements for safety and health standards in places of employment. Fines for noncompliance can be steep.

6. **Resale permits.**

Every person engaged in the business of selling tangible personal property must apply to the state tax office for a seller's permit. This would apply to nutritional supplements legally saleable to patients. If you use herbs during the time of treatment and their use is part of your treatment fee, this would not constitute 'sale of tangible property'.

Where To Practice

The Geographic Area

> **Suggestion:** Use the check mark boxes as you select your location. Does your location have all of the advantages you want? Check mark the advantages of your location in blue or black pen. Check mark the disadvantages which are of concern to you in red.

Discovering where to locate your practice can be a great adventure. You'll be thinking about the kind of activities in which you want to become involved and the kind of scenery you want . It's the time when you are thinking about your dream and about making your practice a success!

One big ingredient of your success is location. If you have ever known a realtor, you will hear the cry: "Location! Location! Location!" It's one resource which can be one of your greatest assets. The other side of the coin is that it could also be your greatest liability. So it's worth it to spend a small amount of quality time investigating what will affect the rest of your time in months and years to come.

When you think of locating or relocating, you not only set up or reset your practice, but you establish yourself in that new location. Some places take a shorter time than others to establish yourself. And when you are starting a practice with limited funds, this can be critical to your success. Certain kinds of areas and sites are easier to start or build your practice because people can afford to come to you, your specialty attracts that area very easily, and people are educated or easily educable to what you do. Your adventure is to find that special place where you can be happy, successful with your patients, and prosper.

❑ *First, start by visualizing a place you want to be.*

Visualize being in the scenery you want to experience, the type of climate, and the activities in which you want to be involved. Is that a place where you can be happy? Is freedom from possible environmental struggle important to you? Is your possible choice by the ocean, the mountains, or a lake? In the big city, the country, or suburbia? Near your family, your relatives, your current friends? Near your normal recreation, near cultural events, near a place that reminds you of where you grew up? Near a research center?

Where ever you choose, find a place you can put your best into your practice. If you choose a place where you know practices do well and you don't want to be there, you won't be able to put 100% of you into your practice. If your dream is to be going to the ocean for a run on a warm beach every day after work, and you settle inland or in a cold area, you won't be happy. You will be thinking about when you move to the place where you want to be—by that warm ocean. If you choose a place you love, but the population base is too small to support your practice, or the population is too stuck to accept acupuncture, you may find yourself struggling to make ends meet. Being on the beach won't be as much fun because you'll be thinking about how and if you will make the rent. So think it through carefully.

❑ *Next explore: 'What state or country would best fit what I want and do best?'*

The legal location will determine how much freedom you have to practice what you want to practice. Laws in that state or country can determine not only the regulations for licensure, including your training, and what and under whom you must practice, but also govern the regulations of insurance, which is the bread and butter of many health care practices.

Some states and countries are more pro-acupuncture than others. The Traditional Acupuncture Institute in Maryland, U.S. has published a booklet describing who to contact in each U.S. state regarding requirements. The California Acupuncture Alliance has published information on this as well. Check with the state board or licensing board in the state or country you are exploring. Listen to their attitude, obtain their rules and regulations, and ask the number of licensed acupuncturists in that state or country.

You may need to take an additional licensing examination to be qualified in a different state or country.

Some states reciprocate with other states. Some states do not . Training in another country may or may not be applicable to your obtaining licensure in the area you are pursuing. If your training was recorded in a different language, this may cause delays in obtaining licensure. If you do need to take another exam or further training to take an exam, find out how long the whole procedure takes before you know you are qualified to practice in that state. Prepare well enough in advance. Some graduates prefer to study and take additional exams close together while the exam material is still fresh for them. You'll want to know you have passed the exam in another state *before* you move there.

❑ ***Get additional feedback. Survey other practitioners.***

Do you know anyone whom you could contact in the state or area you are considering? Perhaps another practitioner in your field who lives there. This you could find out through the Referral Directory of your local or national health professional association. Speaking with other acupuncturists in the area you are considerations can give you insightful information about the success of similar practices started in their area.

❑ ***Research the need for your service.***

In a service business, your service potential will depend on the area you serve. How many potential patients in the area will need your services? Is it an area educated to your services? Or will it require extensive education? Is there an openness to acupuncture?

One way to determine if there is a need for your services in an area and the best possibility of being profitable is to do a survey yourself. This can build a connection with future patients in the area that will reap extensive financial rewards in the future. I have included two survey questionnaires for your use: 1) "*Demographics and Psychographics on Potential Patients*" and 2) an area survey of like businesses. These are in the next section on "Market Planning." Use the latter questionnaire with health practitioners in the area to network with them.

Personal contact is the best way you can find out how responsive people in an area are to you. Door to door survey may not be your style. However, you may want to get a feel for a selection of the local area homes to see what the local response is. Introduce yourself to local residents and business people, and let people know you are surveying the area because you are considering opening an acupuncture practice in their immediate area. Ask them if they or their family has ever been treated successfully with acupuncture. If yes, give them your card, build rapport, and ask them if they would like you to contact them when you open your practice in their neighborhood. Be sure you keep a list of those follow-ups. They can be your initial marketing thrust.

If the people you contact don't know about acupuncture, ask they if they have had any condition they are concerned about. If yes, let them know if you treat this condition. If you believe you can assist them, tell them. Tell them you will send them a booklet on "Questions and Answers about Acupuncture" [1] (and a pamphlet on their condition if you have any), and you will be happy to contact them as soon as you have an office. If you do home calls, tell them. Obtain their name, phone number, and address. We don't recommend treatment on the spot. It can generally appear unprofessional. Follow-up with a phone call and set an appointment as soon as possible.

❑ You may find it valuable to use a map to pinpoint where the health practitioners are in the towns you are considering. Put dots on the map for the practitioners who offer your services. Are these locations successful?

❑ *Get clear and decide whether you want to practice in a metropolitan, suburban or rural area.*

This doesn't mean you have to live in the same area in which you practice. You may want to commute. Consider:

■ 1. Population and its growth potential.
■ 2. Income, age, occupation, and type of population.
■ 3. Local ordinances and zoning regulations.
■ 4. Type of trading area (commercial, industrial, residential, seasonal).
■ 5. The success and number of competitive services in and around your proposed locations.

Advantages of a city practice are:
■ 1. More availability of patients.
■ 2. Larger pool of people to choose from, with many professionals who may refer patients to you.
■ 3. Large institutions/schools in which to teach.

Advantages of a rural practice are:
■ 1. It's a smaller population with greater opportunity to know the people of the town personally.
■ 2. A quieter, less stressful life for you and your patients.
■ 3. Being in more aesthetic, natural, unpolluted surroundings.
■ 4. It's less expensive and requires less overhead to run than a city practice.

[1] "Questions and Answers About Acupuncture" is part of the 8 pamphlet series available From Tao to Earth, Focus Practice Management Publications Distribution at 1 (800) 800-3139.

(If you do practice in a rural town or small town, located right in the middle of town, not out on a rural route road.)

❑ *Concerning the population and growth, you want to be in an area that is growing.*

Check the population ten years ago to what it is now. This will give you the percentage of growth for the town. Contact the Chamber of Commerce in the town(s) you choose and determine the ratio of population to acupuncturists in these towns, and the ratio of acupuncturists to other health practitioners in the town. A ratio of one acupuncturist to 10,000 population is good, but a ratio of 1 to 35,000 people is better. Go where you are needed. Right now probably the highest concentration of acupuncturists are near where the acupuncture colleges are located and in the larger metropolitan cities.

❑ *Look for a well established town where people place added value on their health and consider what happens if they are without it.*
This more often falls with the range of 45-55+ year old people. This may also include populations of people who go specifically to a town or locale renown for its healthy climate and atmosphere, its health consciousness, and its innovative practitioners. Remember, that all ages may be attracted to you. However, specific age brackets are more economically stable and can stabilize your practice. Older people generally are more stable occupation-wise, financially and live in one place longer, so may come to you with greater consistency over a longer period of time. The age bracket of the people surrounding an office (and what goes with the age) has made a crucial difference in many practitioners' success or failure. Don't be fooled by new moderate to below moderate housing (which may be well-mortgaged or rented). Look for what is established surrounding you. Just make sure your financial base is covered from a business standpoint.

❑ *Future Growth.*
What current building is going on? New banks, grocery stores, real estate booming? Is there a strong economic base? Are nearby industries working full time? Only part time? Did any industries go out of business in the past several months? Is the town dependent on one industry? (If the industry is on strike, the whole town will be out of work). Make sure there is plenty of work present to support your practice.

❏ *Low turnover neighborhood.*
Make sure you are in an area that is committed to quality care—where the buildings are painted, repaired and landscaped nicely. If you are in a changing neighborhood where there is a high turnover of renters such as in a college town neighborhood; or in a government low income housing area, the commitment to keeping up the property and paying their bills may be lower.

❏ *What is the ethnic and socioeconomic pattern of the town?*
It may be to your advantage, for example, if you are Chinese and settle in a predominately Chinese area because of the clannish support of an ethnic group. However, it may work against you if you are considered an "outsider", particularly in small towns or cliquish neighborhoods.

❏ *Also, unless you want to be on a state program, you may not want to settle in the middle of a thousand welfare recipients. See what fits and feels comfortable to you.*

❏ *Growth Zone.*
Make sure the property you are buying is in a growth area. Not only will your practice grow, but your property value will increase.

While we often tend to choose an area because it "feels right," (and we may not have an explanation for this), it helps to open our vision and hone our perceptions of the area we are considering practicing. We'll be looking at the people and their needs in the next section, as well as why you would choose a particular kind of office site (pp. 180-7).

These points were cited from Dr. Peter Fernandez's book, *How to Start a Profitable Practice from Scratch,* 1980, and the SBA pamphlet, *"Starting and Managing a Small Business of Your Own."*

REACHING YOUR PATIENTS

How to Develop Your Marketing Plan

> ### The Seven Essentials of a Health Care Marketing Plan
> 1. Identify your potential market – new patients, best patient referrers, and practitioner referral network.
> 2. Define your marketing approach: service concept, special skills and areas of expertise, image, and your unique advantage.
> 3. Contact your potential market.
> 4. Convey the benefit and uniqueness of your service.
> 5. Communicate how you can fill their need.
> 6. Convey a sense of urgency in getting their needs fulfilled.
> 7. Meet the practice short and long range objectives: Create a commitment to come to the office, follow-through with care, get well, pay, return if an old or new problem occurs, and refer others.

Reaching Potential Patients in Today's Market

A priority consideration in successful practice is finding the *best* way to reach your potential patients. Successfully reaching your potential patients will require forethought, planning, and the following: 1) demographics and psychographics (market research) on the areas health care market, 2) what is called "packaging" – the way you and your practice are presented and 3) the right use of media to best reach your specific new patient base.

Many service organizations never take the time to consider *who* they can best reach and *what kind* of presentation would best reach them. Hence, many fail. Market research on potential patients in your location of choice will tell you what kind of reception you will be dealing with, what motivates your potential patients, as well as what the supply and demand is in the area. This is part of knowing how to present yourself to your market. The other part is designing your "service concept" (or health care package), presenting yourself, and then influencing through the best means available.

A "service concept" is composed of the following answers to these questions. So get out your pen and consider these: What do you offer? What do you do compared to what people think you do? What does your potential patient market prefer in a health care practice? How can you communicate more clearly what you actually do? What kind of atmosphere will you provide? What can you do to stand out or be extraordinary? How will you create becoming "preferred" in your market? What can you offer to invite the patient to try your services? Why will they return?

What will they need in three months, six months, a year, when their present needs have been met? What can you offer that no one else can? These all go into your image and the type of practice you have. These are questions that must be answered to make an effective marketing plan.

Most practitioners truly want to reach out to their potential patients. However, many have not known how to *describe* their "service concept" and have simply been disgusted and turned off to marketing itself because of the amount of gimmicks, sensationalism, and poor ethics used in marketing and advertising, as well as abused referral building practices. We have all seen marketing in the business world which has been focused around getting action at all costs, rather than creating connectedness and promoting positive action. However, people do respond favorably to certain types of marketing and advertising in the health care field, and they will respond to what is believable. They do respond on a feeling tone level to what they sense has integrity, a tone of caring, and will benefit them. A good "service concept" which matches the needs of the targeted area is a real key to successful marketing.

Realities of Marketing in the Medical Field

The attitude in the medical profession is fast changing regarding marketing and advertising. Many practitioners, clinics, and hospitals are recognizing the importance and need to create a preference for their services, amidst the full range of health care services offered today. Many of their ads and marketing techniques are taking into consideration what the needs and wants of their potential patients are, and they are presenting an image which can be backed up by good care. They are bringing a warmer, genuine tone to the market place. They are learning to use media in a way which reaches people where they are.

In this day and age, the world of health care is waking up to the fact that success goes to those who understand and use media effectively. It's the practitioner's choice to understand media and use them rightly *or* disdain them and limit his options for growth and expansion.

Safe practice, rapport, and the reputation lay a foundation for reaching potential patients. These are all elements of good presentation. However, first: 1) understand your market, 2) find out *facts* which make a good location and service match, 3) show others – particularly your specific niche – how you can benefit them, 4) do planned marketing and advertising, and 5) do planned referral building. These are the *keys* to both reach new patients and develop a "steady" referral base. So this section will be devoted to these areas.

Identifying Your Potential Patients

Practitioners who succeed fill a specific need in their community. As we mentioned earlier, there must be a need and demand for your talents, tendencies, and service in your area of choice. Once you determine this, you can then identify who your potential patients will be and what they want. After this step, the objective is to create a "preference" for your services in your location.

Who will be your primary source of clients -- or your "target market?" This begins with market research. The most successful way of getting a market profile is through demographics and psychographics. Demographics tell you who your patients are, where *your* specialty's population is, and where to find those people. Psychographics tell you what and why they will choose your services.

Demographics

Demographic studies provide statistical information about your potential patients, describing them by age, income, education, sex, health problems, months of higher incidence of specific health conditions, things that help you to identify them as a specific segment of the population. It can also tell you information about climate in the area, and how it impacts the people environmentally and health-wise.

Probably the **best** source for your inquiry is probably the Department of Health (county and/or state) in the area you are considering. You can find out the health statistics in many locations for different ages, socioeconomic backgrounds, months of specific illnesses, and what the health needs of that area are.

Other demographic research can be done at public or university libraries where you will find statistics compiled by the city, county, state and U.S. government. The Chamber of Commerce is an excellent source of demographic data -- on large self-insured employers, for example. You may want this information to investigate what companies have physician teams. You could then do research on how you might be recommended by those teams for workers' compensation cases.

Find out everything you can about your potential patients that will help you reach them and motivate them to be your patient. Identify your patient by health problem, month of high incidence of illness, age, address, income, employment, etc. Magazines and newspapers specific to the area will give you a feeling for the attitude of various sectors of the population in the area.

If your practice focuses on blood diseases, coronary heart disease, and blood pressure screenings, where will you find a high incidence of people who will need and can afford your services? Settling in a low income Medicare neighborhood where people can't afford your services wouldn't be your top location choice. Neither would a neighborhood predominately made up of young families with children. A medical complex near a hospital with a middle to higher income clientele and a strong potential base for physician referrals might be the key for you. What months are there higher incidences of illness? After discovering these demographics, consider how would you promote prevention, relief, stabilization, optimal care, and maintenance care to your target group.

Find out about the climate and seasons and how this affects the health of your potential patients. This will help you determine when to market and for what conditions.

If you have a specialty or subspecialty in allergies, you may want to look for a location that has a high incidence of air-pollution or seasonal allergy-producing pollen in the air. The best advertising will promote 1) good personal service 2) pain free treatments (acupuncture doesn't hurt like shots often do) and 3) repeat business. (Have the patient fill out a self-addressed reminder card in seasons when the pollen count is high).

If allergies are a subspecialty, market to your potential patients in seasons in which this condition is prevalent. If colds and flu-prevention are a specialty, market this in the month preceding those which are seasonally flu and cold prone months.

Psychographics

WHY and WHAT KIND of services the patients will pay for is tougher to determine because it is so subjective. Psychographics describe the patient's attitudes and motivations, tell what patients want to experience from a particular kind of health care approach, and why they will pay for it. To uncover the potential patient's motives, you must put yourself into their shoes. Talk to them. Check out the local newspapers to explore their concerns and interests. See where you would go for a particular condition. Why you would do it? What would you expect? How often would you be willing to go for care? Long treatments? Short treatments? How much would it interfere with work? What would be the best benefit? Acupuncture or related therapy preferences? What would you have to overcome to have acupuncture services? What would you want to know before you received acupuncture services? What would you want to know about the health care provider? What kind of results could you expect? What characteristics would you want in this treating practitioner? What adjuncts would you buy? What would you be willing to pay if you were in their shoes?

You can find out some of this information by going to other services which are condition oriented, such as the American Lung Association, the Cancer Foundation, or the Heart Association, methadone clinics, weight loss clinics. They may be willing to provide you with a mailing list and/or want to employ your services for consultation, referral, or treatment.

Market research institutes (qualitative and quantitative) and/or advertising agencies who have targeted studies on the response of patients in their area may be of assistance. For the latest such marketing information as it relates to your requirements, contact the following syndicated research services directly:

American Research Bureau
4320 Ammendale Road
Beltsville, MD 20705

** Blackstone Group
Contact: Valerie Wohl
360 N. Michigan Ave.
Chicago, IL 60601
(312) 419-0400

Brand Rating Research Corp.
745 Fifth Avenue
New York, NY 10022

Gallup & Robinson, Inc.
44 Nassau Street
Princeton, NY 08541

N. C. Rorabaugh Co., Inc.
347 Madison Avenue
New York, NY 10017
--
W. R. Simmons & Associates
Research, Incorporated
235 East 42nd Street
New York, NY 10017

Sindlinger & Co., Inc.
Winona & Mohawk Avenues
Norwood, PA 19074

SRDS Data, Inc.
235 East 42nd Street
New York, NY 10017

C. E. Hooper, Inc.
750 Third Avenue
New York, NY 10017

A.C. Nielsen Company
1290 Avenue of the Americas
New York, NY 10019

Alfred Politz Research, Inc.
527 Madison Avenue
New York, NY 10022

The Pulse, Inc.
730 Fifth Avenue
New York, NY 10019

Trendex, Inc.
200 Park Avenue
New York, NY 10017

Yankelovich, Skelly & White, Inc.
969 High Ridge Road
Stamford, CT 06905

Daniel Starch and Staff
Mamaroneck, NY 10544

For further information on demographics in your specific area, direct mail distributors usually do studies on the market.

It would also be wise to check on the competition (see survey in this section) to see how they are marketing their practices. What advertising are they doing in the area? How many competitors are there who do what you do? No matter how good you are, how well you manage your patient's experience of you, or how good you make the patient feel, if there is too much competition in the area, your business has a much lesser chance of success. Your survey could make the difference!

**At the time of this writing, Blackstone Group was doing a research study for acupuncture practices in the U.S.

Demographics and Psychographics

Keep your objectives and basic goals in mind. REMEMBER, goals are specific in time commitment and degree of commitment. Use your research on the demographics and psychographics to help you fill your goals and objectives.

Example Objectives

Moral objective: To bring the healing world of acupuncture to as many people as possible.

Business objective: To make a fair and reasonable profit.

Marketing objective: To create a demand for your services.

Advertising objective: To create a preference for your services.

1. MORAL Goal:
2. BUSINESS Goal:
3. MARKETING Goal:
4. ADVERTISING Goal:

WHAT AREA geographically will you target your marketing? _____
_____
_____

WHO are your target market persons? (Check with the Health Department, library, etc. Speak to individuals.)

1. Major Health problem(s) _____
2. Month/season of health problem(s): _____
3. Permanent, transient: _____
4. Married, unmarried: _____
5. Age bracket: _____
6. Income: _____
7. Occupation: _____
8. Life style: _____
9. Children: _____
10. Families, women, or men specifically: _____
11. Ethnic background: _____

1.   Secondary Health problem(s): _____
2.   Month/season of health problem(s): _____
3.   Permanent, transient: _____
4.   Married, unmarried: _____
5.   Age bracket: _____
6.   Income: _____
7.   Occupation: _____
8.   Life style: _____
9.   Children: _____
10.   Families, women or men specifically: _____
11.   Ethnic background: _____

1.   Other health problem(s): _____
2.   Month/season of health problem(s): _____

1.   Other health problem(s): _____
2.   Month/season of health problem(s): _____

WHERE DO THEY LIVE?

1)   Suburban, middle-income tract development _____
2)   Middle-income urban renewal area _____
3)   Rural area _____
4)   Downtown area _____
5)   Middle to wealthy area _____
5)   Wealthy area _____
6)   Working class lower income area _____
7)   Within ten miles of your practice _____

What kind of services do they now go to in order to receive similar health services?

_____
_____

Where are they located?

_____

Is this a preferred area?

_____

Is there a preferred area where services aren't being offered to your targeted market? _____

WHY will they pay for these services? Rank priorities and comment.

1. Expertise in specific specialty _____
2. Best available. _____
3. Degree they want good results _____
4. Tried everything else; willing to try acupuncture _____

5. Good reputation even though little understanding of acupuncture _____

6. Relief care _____
7. Total health care planning _____
8. Want pain relief _____
9. Best preventative care _____
10. Convenience _____
11. Type of location _____
12. Time saving _____
13. Young, progressive practitioner _____
14. Older experienced practitioner _____
15. Preference already established in area for acupuncture services _____
16. Preference being established in area for alternative health care service. _____
17. Openness to new health care services. _____
   _____
18. Openness by physicians in the area to refer to acupuncturists.
   _____

For **WHAT** services will they pay and **HOW MUCH?** (Free, low cost, medium, higher range)

1. Consultation: _____
2. Examination and acupuncture treatment: _____
3. Related therapies:
   _____
   _____
   _____
4. Type of adjuncts:
   Magnetic jewelry _____
   Magnetic supports, pad, seat, discs _____
   Other supports _____
   Herbs _____
   Nutritional supplements _____

What's your **UNIQUE ADVANTAGE** in your demographic and geographic area?_____

_____

_____

_____

_____

_____

HOW DO YOU BEST REACH your patients with your message in a cost effective way?_____

_____

_____

Where do you go to interact with your target market?_____

_____

_____

Where do they usually go to most obviously find out about the type of service you offer?_____

_____

_____

_____

Where do you read about them to keep abreast of their life style, health styles, their community? _____

_____

What newspapers, magazines, notices, do they read to find out about who
you are, what acupuncture is, how it benefits them, etc.?

_____

_____

_____

_____

_____

_____

_____

_____

_____

Area Survey
Assessing the Need and Demand for Your Services

Where is the Competition? Your Complements? Your Niche?

> Research your information by using the phone books in your library, writing to specific acupuncture colleges, surveying the desired area population, or communicating with the local Chamber of Commerce where you are considering locating. The chamber has statistical and demographic information. Talk with the local allied professionals and research the questions below.

1. How many acupuncturists are there in the area?_____

2. How many closely allied practitioners handle your service?____

3. What is their view on the advantages of their location?_____

   _____

   _____

   _____

   _____

   _____

   _____

   _____

   _____

4. Do they want to network?_____ Associate?_____ Refer? ____

5. Is the area saturated with acupuncturists? ____

   With natural healers ____health professionals generally? _____

6. Is there an area that is booming and has a need for more practitioners such as yourself?_____ Where?

   _____

   _____

   _____

7. How many of these professionals look prosperous?_____

8. Do they have apparent advantages over you?_____ What?
    _____
    _____
    _____
    _____

9. How many are barely getting by?_____

10. How many similar services went out of business in the area in the

    last year?_____Why?_____
    _____
    _____

11. How many similar services opened up in the last year?_____

12. How much do they charge for services that you provide? _____
    _____
    _____

13. Which practices will be your biggest competitors? _____
    _____

    Why? _____
    _____

14. What unique advantage do you offer? (Specialties, equipment,
    values, type of services, what you do better, more of, differently, etc.)
    _____
    _____
    _____
    _____
    _____

15. What services in demand do you not offer? _____
    _____
    _____

16. How can you complement the services of other allied practitioners?
    _____
    _____
    _____
    _____

After reviewing these questions, do you still want to practice "on your own", or work in conjunction with an allied practitioner?

Scope of Practice and Service Concept

Even though you may be in the midst of career choice or study in one approach, consider the impact of combined approaches together. Those combined approaoches may determine what you can and cannot do with patients, as well as the direction, ease and type of growth, type of patients, and income producing ability from insurance or patients. You may want to consider your scope of practice in relationship to the area in which you want to practice when making your choice of health care approach.

Choices which can be combined:

Acupuncturist
Oriental Medical Doctor
WITH
Specialty_____
Medical Doctor
Medicalspecialty _____
Herbalist
Nutritionist
Herbalist

Naturopath
Homeopathatic Physician
Chiropractic Physician
Osteopathic Physician
Physical Therapist
Massage Therapist
 Psychotherapist
Other _____
(Legally dependent on state and country)

Write down your Service Concept: (See page 76)

Defining Your Specialty and Unique Advantage

Within the practice of acupuncture are "preferred specialties" which you can use to focus your tendencies, your market advantage, and give people a way of defining you. Defining a specialty does not mean that you have to limit your abilities. A specialty choice is not necessarily the only service you provide. Since it is difficult to promote a practice by being all things to all people, you will want to focus on at least one or two specific areas. From the standpoint of practice, this is referred to as targeted markets.

Take a few minutes to consider the specialties listed below. Choose three specific areas you prefer in promoting your practice. If you have a different choice than those listed, include it in the blank space. If you have trouble deciding, perhaps you need to do more research. One way to narrow your choices is to eliminate the areas you will not consider or feel uneasy about. You feel neutral or strong about he remaining ones. What are your strong choices?

Medical incurables specialist
Chronic pain relief specialist
Chronic illnesses
    --non life threatening
    --life threatening
Terminal illness within 6 months
Terminal illness within five years
Degenerative disease
Family medicine - colds, flu,
    preventative care
Pediatric (children) specialist
Geriatric (elderly) specialist
Gynecology specialist
Child birth specialist
Women's specialist
Men's specialist -- hair disorders,
    impotence, illness & injury, etc.
Functional illnesses _____
Workers' injury practitioner
Personal injury practitioner
Insurance practice

Blood diseases and cardiac problems
    blood pressure screenings
Gastrointestinal / Internal specialist
Skin rejuvenation & face lift specialist
Allergy and skin disorder specialist
Nutritional specialist
Specialty testing for _____
    Athletic injury specialist
Counseling specialty (area) _____
Health education
Beauty specialist
Dental specialist
Veterinary specialist
Headache specialist
Addiction specialist
    --weight control
    --detoxification
    --stop smoking etc.
    --drug rehabilitation
Psychic illnesses, trauma
Post operative pain specialist
Other_____

Unique Advantage _____

_____

_____

Type of Practice

The *type* of practice you have defines how you expect people to see you. It creates your image and adds to your service concept. It becomes your "unique advantage" as it fits the location where you choose to practice.

The following combinations are ways you can show and describe what you are about. Check which approach you will take:

- ❏ Scope of practice (page 87)
- ❏ Emphasis on women, men, babies, young children, adolescents, elderly
- ❏ Specialty (s) conditions vs. generalized (listed on page 88)
- ❏ Personal vs. impersonal care
- ❏ Emphasis on diagnostic abilities and equiipment, treatment abilities, or both
- ❏ Relief care vs. educating and treating beyond relief
- ❏ Quick care vs. depth of care
- ❏ Emphasis on recommendations, home care, directions, health education vs. none or very little
- ❏ Small vs. large clinic
- ❏ Low-cost clinic vs. extra service clinic
- ❏ Quick paced vs. slower pace
- ❏ Long waits for care vs. on time practice
- ❏ Multiple practitioners vs. single practitioner
- ❏ Traditional methods vs. mixed treatment methods
- ❏ Wholistic health care clinic vs. standard medical clinic
- ❏ Preferred provider clinic vs. non preferred provider private practice
- ❏ Hospital practice
- ❏ On call practice
- ❏ Work injury or accidental injury emphasis
- ❏ Small town intimate homespun practice image
- ❏ Modernized medical complex image
- ❏ Ethnic "Chinatown" image
- ❏ Conservative vs. non-conservative practice
- ❏ Progressive vs. fixed ways

Remember: <u>Patient's perceive you and your practice as a whole package</u>. Make sure your tone and type of practice fits your demographic and psychographic location. Then your ability to communicate your attitude and type of practice clearly can attract new patients and help them communicate who you are and what you are about to others. So plan your practice as a whole package, including your practice image, so they can see that you are their "preferred" choice. **List your unique advantages.** These will help you market.

How to Reach Out to Your Market and Handle Response

Practitioners must be time and cost-conscious in marketing. Look at what efforts bring the greatest return. To use your time profitably, don't bother to initiate something you can't or won't follow-up on. Otherwise, you will abort your efforts. Follow-up is essential in marketing. Spend your dollars well in a few strategic places.

1. **Put your name, address, and phone number in local phone and medical referral directories** so people can access you. Include qualifications, specialties, modalities, etc.

2. Hire a trained front office manager who will be your best **referral promoter.** He/she should handle all inquiries well on the phone, and be knowledgeable about health care promotion. This should someone who is willing to expand your office and will use methods to keep his/her enthusiasm alive. The dialogues, promotion and education procedure in *Volume II* are excellent for this purpose.

   Your front office assistant should be able to handle calls from new patients artfully. Any marketing you do will fail if he or she can't promote you with assurance or doesn't have the knack of finding ways to assuage the patient's reservations. This is why telephone promotion ability is so vital. Good phone presentation is essential in handling patient response.

3. **ASK for referrals** from friends and colleagues. Don't be overly proud. You want your friends and patients to know that you would like to build your practice. Write down specific names to write, call, or follow-up.

4. Keep your focus on **serving people.** Always have a small **appointment book** with you, as well as **appointment cards.** Before you leave the office, note the times you want to fill. Be receptive to people's needs anywhere you go. Be willing to serve them. Be courageous enough to walk up to a stranger you see in pain and say, "I am _____,an acupuncturist (or doctor of Oriental Medicine.) I think I may be able to help you. Call me at my office. I would be happy to give you a courtesy consultation." Give them your card with the phone number on it. If the person expresses immediate interest, talk to them briefly. Don't do the consultation then! Schedule the appointment on the spot.

5. Keep your focus on **networking for referrals**. When you go to medical or hospital functions, meet others interested in what you do. Speak with M.D.s who specialize in fields appropriate to your target market. Develop a referral base.

   Educate other practitioners on what you do. Many have a number of questions or simply don't know enough about the benefits of acupuncture. It is important to follow-up on these interested contacts and develop them! Give the practitioners whatever information they need to learn more about what you do, how it will benefit them in referring, and follow-up any reports you send by phone. You must establish a comfortable working relationship before they will refer to you initially and continue to refer.

6. **Meet people who refer to practitioners:** gym directors, coaches, group employers, specialized doctors and lawyers who work (for example) with workers' compensation cases. Use the seven essentials of your marketing plan.

   In considering how you can fill their needs, be prepared. When you address self-insured employers, you must be able to convey your knowledge, such as statistics on acupuncture care's effectiveness and cost-savings in areas western medicine can't compete.

7. **Arrange to have a presentation** if you enjoy speaking or have good demonstration skills . It is important to have people sign in with their phone number and address when they enter. In your speech convey benefits of care, urgency in handling health condition(s), and give incentives to make an appointment at the end of session for individual consultation. Do follow-up calls to assure patient follow-through. In the beginning of practice, a trained front office person should have the expertise and time to make these calls. This is an investment in your future.

8. **Put your picture and a weekly or monthly column** in the newspaper illustrating how acupuncture care relieves a condition targeted for your demographic area. If placed correctly, it can be an effective way to educate your patient base and build your image -- especially if you are unknown.

9. **Place local newspaper ads** targeting conditions in appropriate sections of the paper. Have these evaluated by an advertising

professional in the medical field. See Volume V, Ads for Acupuncturists for examples or ads you are free to use.

10. **Send direct mail** letters to your demographic target group using the seven essentials of your marketing plan (also see **Volume IV**). Check into sending your mailing out "co-op" with a targeted association's newsletter. (For example, if your specialty is diabetes, send it to the local diabetes association or support group.) Follow-up with assistant's phone calls. Practice by using a script for the call to create the results you want.

11. **Use** patient histories with **"former doctor" listed** on the form. Develop your liaison and referral base from calling these doctors regarding their patient. (Make sure you have a "Release of Medical Information" by the patient on file.) To build your referral base, you must communicate that you are getting results with their current patients, communicate how you can fill other gaps for that practitioner, consider what patients might be appropriate to refer to you, and follow-up on these.

12. **"Touch and tell treatment program"** (plus referral building procedure) with Personal Acupuncture Care Report & Recommendations, Patient Care letter, Planned Schedule of Appointments & Reevaluation, Brochure on their condition — and other conditions acupuncture treats successfully reinforces the patient's results and enthusiasm about you.

13. **Acupuncture health care classes.**
When you schedule your patients for an orientation health care class, have them invite their support person and friends. This can open up your market. Offering health care classes in either an adult education program, a treatment care facility, your own facility, or an employer sponsored safety and health care presentation in their facility, can be useful in opening up your market.

14. **Referral-building procedures** (see Patient Visit Procedure section)

15. **Practitioner referral-building procedure** (See next section).

Note: *Volume IV: Patient Communication, Public Relations and Marketing* delves into what marketing methods to use, what makes them effective, and many visual presentations of marketing and advertising which work. *Advertising for Acupuncturists* contains the ads to use. They are grouped to use for specific purposes.

Building a Practitioner Referral Base Network

No matter how competent you are in your field, the practitioner who finds his referral base before giving up in his search comes out ahead. He must have this referral base to build his practice and to refer out areas of patient care for which he is not equipped. An acupuncturist does not have to be all things to all patients to serve safely and competently. No health care practitioner could expect to be. This fact alone compels most to seek a range of other practitioners to refer to. This is only safe practice.

Think about your health care network for a moment, and consider how the following specialties can complement your care for your patients: Western medical doctors. . . What specific fields. . . ? Other Oriental medical practitioners. . . Which areas of expertise . . .? Osteopaths, chiropractors, naturopaths, herbalists, nutritionists, massage therapists, psychotherapists, and others. This is your potential referral network. What is their scope of practice and how can you utilize it . . . ? **Make a list of your potential practitioner base, their fields, and where you can best meet and speak with them. Follow through until you have a good mutual referral base.**

Developing a **strong** referral base is not a sign of weakness. Indeed, it signifies to other practitioners and patients that you have a broader perspective than the limits of your practice. You can avoid malpractice problems by not treating beyond the scope of acupuncture. Referring out appropriately can show that your priority is to see your patients well, not letting pride, ego, and the pocketbook rule your decisions. It can also be used to build your referral base with other practitioners and to educate other practitioners about the care in which you excel. When patient care is your primary consideration, referrals to others with follow-up communication can often lead to referrals to you. Rapport is the key.

New practitioners often connect with other practitioners, whereby nothing comes of the connection. Do not give up. You may have to make a number of initial and follow-up calls or go to several practitioner events before making a solid connection. How you approach potential practitioners regarding referrals will determine if they are interested in developing a rapport with you. Their needs and perspectives at the time are the other factors. Consider the following approach:

1) Be sincere in your concern to provide the best service to your patient.

2) Let the practitioner know you are looking for another professional to whom you can refer patients with different therapy needs than you provide, and who complements your practice.

3) Let him know you are interested in one who is open to the use of acupuncture as a complement to his practice. Inquire about his needs. Let him know how you can meet them. Be frank about your strengths, excellent results in specialty areas, and how your skills can complement his. Find out what *his* specialty is. Educate one another about your fields of expertise, specific conditions, etc.

Make connections with health care practitioners by attending (or giving) lectures in your local area on topics of special interest to them. You can inform others of new information in the field and meet other practitioners who could become valuable allies. This is a good time to talk about how you can serve each other. At these events they already have in mind the intention of exploring other avenues of health care. Referral networking is one of them.

Another way to increase rapport with other practitioners is to keep current by reading magazines on breakthroughs in the health care field. You will know who and what kind of conditions will respond with the new technology and research available, and may want to connect with the practitioners in your area involved in this field.

A new patient coming to your practice offers you the opportunity to contact his former or concurring physician and develop a rapport with him. It may be appropriate to ask your patient to have his medical records sent to you for review. Let your patient know if it is beneficial for you to communicate with his medical doctor. If this is agreeable to the patient, this is an excellent way of building a liaison for future referrals. With the patient's permission, offer to send the physician a report of your findings when appropriate. Keep up communication with other practitioners with whom you have mutual care patients, and send them clear reports on your patients.

The keys to referral building: Rapport and mutual confidence in one another. Other professionals will notice your sincerity and desire to give excellent patient care — including the ability to find the *right* referral for a specific condition.

YOUR REPUTATION AND IMAGE

Creating Reputation and Building Image

One of the first questions I am often asked about reputation is, "Why do I need an image to build reputation?" The fact is that every person and practice *has* an image, whether he realizes it or not. Reputation is built on the attitudes and perceptions that others have about us, regardless of how we perceive ourselves or our practice.

How does this happen? An image consists of attitudes and opinions one has about a person, a practice, or ourselves. These attitudes are formed by impressions and perceptions about that person or practice. The image we have of ourselves is often not the same as the one others perceive. We are not usually conscious of this; however, we are reminded when we receive feedback from our environment regarding our behavior. If the feedback is positive, we are pleased and feel there is no need to improve. However, because thinking tends to be selective, we may overlook areas that need improvement. On the other hand if the feedback is negative, we feel obliged to change something in our behavior to equate our self-image with the outside-image we convey. We feel particularly compelled to improve if the feedback comes from people we value and respect. The same process applies with your practice.

Frequently practitioners are so intent on their attitude and approach towards patients that they blind themselves to the image patients receive about other aspects of the practice. They may not see how staff attitudes toward patient care and procedure affect their clientele, how patient omissions affect their practice, or how the right location and front office appearance influences their patients' attitudes. Patients may like their practitioner, but feel cool toward the practice. The result is either a lower referral rate or referral of patient types who have specific characteristics or conditions which you do not want to promote. We must consciously ask, obtain, and listen to feedback from staff, patients, and the public in monitoring ourselves and our practices.

We know from psychological studies that images form on the emotional level, not necessarily on the cognitive one. Therefore it is important for your patients to get the right "gut feeling" when they walk into your practice or talk to your assistant on the phone. Of course, information also constitutes an image; therefore make sure you present your patients with information you want them to remember about you.

We emphasize image because in the beginning of your practice, you start from "neutral ground", i.e. without an image. Once an image has been established it is very hard to change it — particularly in the positive direction. Depending on which actions you take, you and your staff can ruin <u>or</u> build your image!

We emphasize image so strongly because in the beginning of your practice, you start from "neutral ground", i.e. without an image. Once an image has been established it is very hard to change it—particularly in the positive direction. Depending on which actions you take, you and your staff can ruin or build your important image!

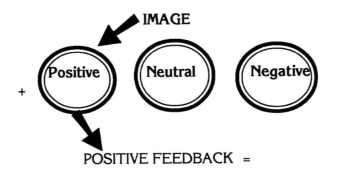

POSITIVE FEEDBACK =

Balanced Patient Turnover	**N**ew Patient Response from Advertising
Returning Former Patients	Low Collection Problems
High Referrals	Favorable Acupuncture Legislatiion
Steady Patient Volume	Payment by Insurance Companies

So how do you build reputation and convey the image you want to project?

■ Convey safe practice, competency, and rapport — both with your patients and to other practitioners. This is the crux of acceptance by patients and other practitioners alike. Follow-up with your patients and your practitioner referral base with care and concern.

■ Look carefully at your service concepts, values, and objectives; the way you communicate them; and how you want to project them. Refer to the sections in this book that address this specifically.

■ Demonstrate how you intend to be successful with patients by using a number of means, including touch, treatment planning, explanation of expectations and benefits, audiovisual aids, etc.

■ Hire a competent staff that can communicate your intentions and objectives clearly and who provide the extra attention that creates patient enthusiasm and loyalty.

■ Set consistent and reasonable office policy and inspire your staff to carry it out.

■ Conscientiously communicate benefits, dedication, and professionalism in referral-building procedures.

■ Show your professionalism in the appearance of your office. It should be inclusive, inspiring and harmonious; organized; bright, fresh, and inviting; comfortable, accommodating, and up-to-date. It should be acceptable to those patients you want to attract. These impression create a credible image!

■ Reach out. Invite referrals from your patients. Participate in the community. Advertise to whom you want to attract.

<u>These are the objectives and top priorities of successful practice.</u>

Reputation and Safe Practice

The following image is the foundation of your personal reputation and the reputation of acupuncture.

> *"The public is in safe and competent hands with you."*

Aside from the fears of change and the ensuing consequences, a reactionary fear around safe practice has caused politically oriented organizations to go to great lengths to limit professions which they do not either understand or believe to have a developed enough overview or methodology to practice either safely or stay within the scope of their licensure. Hence, regardless of other roles, in the role of public defender, the approach is with reserve, caution, and protection.

It takes time, planning, and willingness to build acceptance and reputation, either as an individual practitioner, or as part of a profession which is little known or understood. As an acupuncturist and oriental medical practitioner, it is your privilege to educate the public and existing practitioners about you as an acupuncturist and acupuncture as a complementary profession.

Build and educate upon the premise or belief that the public is in safe and competent hands with you. Continually back this up in fact. As this is so, you will be in position to touch more people with your gift. A safe practice reputation--your and acupuncture's--can be one of your biggest assets.

The following are areas of reputation and image building:

- Practitioner's field, specialty, and marketing niche
- Practice presentation
- Treatment rationale, health care planning and projection of attitude
- Quality of staff and staff development
- Safe practice communication and procedures
- Appropriate location for your niche market
- Professional office appearance, conveying your particular uniqueness.
- Quality forms and literature which promote patient care, various levels of health care planning, referral building, your other policies
- Well-thought out fees
- Clear workable financial policies which open options for follow-through care.
- Concern for patient response and feedback.

Who you hire and the level of his/her commitment and development will determine your practice's reputation based on:

- Uplifting patient rapport
- Referral-inspiring communications
- Follow-through patient procedure
- New patient telephone procedures, recalls, and backsliding prevention
- Clear multiple appointment scheduling and appointment book procedure
- Patient orientation and education
- Efficient billing and reporting procedure
- Ease in office flow and organization procedure
- Caring intake and efficient records procedure
- Quality and effective collection procedure
- Quality insurance assistance and procedure

These are worth goals to ensure reputable and successful practice!

The Acupuncturist's Presentation

Practitioners often don't realize that just because they don't have a poor reputation doesn't mean they have a good one. In fact, having no reputation, and therefore no image, is almost like a person without a face. How would you describe such a person? You would probably lack adjectives. The same thing applies to you and your practice if you don't build a profile — something that separates you from your other colleagues, your unique advantage! You may not see why you aren't getting referrals.

The following are some "neutral and discomforting" perceptions which patients have about practitioners and their practices which keep them from recommending a practitioner or referring others. We've also offered some solutions to these problems.

- *No reputation, unknown.*
  Patients have to get through their fear of the unknown, and their fear of being in incompetent hands. They want to be needed, wanted, heard, and helped. If they don't know anything about you, they won't risk. They want to go to someone 1) whom they have either heard of by a friend who had good results, rapport, and prefers this practitioner, 2) by recommendation of an authority, such as another trusted practitioner 3) whom they have heard and seen personally via a lecture or demonstration, 4) whom they have seen a picture and read his words, such as in a newspaper column, 5) about whom they have read in an article, such as in a journal, newspaper, or specialty

publication, 6) who motivates them by the tone and picture in an ad or radio spot, 7) whom they have heard speak personally on the radio or TV. This means that to reach people, they will need marketing efforts such as these and others, so they can get to know you.

A front office assistant who has good public relations skills, and uses the tone and dialog outlined in **Volume II**, can bridge any gulf on that first phone call, so patients feel compelled to come to you. She/he is the bridge between the known and the unknown. From there, she/he sets the tone of the way patient and practice policy and procedures are carried out to serve your patients which can profoundly influence your practice image and reputation.

- *Outdated.*
  Patients want to go to a practitioner who is experienced, but not ignorant of current procedures. For middle class or higher, "old" does not always equal better. In more progressive countries, there is a respect of modern technology in a practitioner. This is an important value to them. These socioeconomic groups want to see practitioners who have updated offices, attitudes, continuing education diplomas on their walls, and equipment — and they are willing to pay the price for those added values.

  Editor's note: No amount of current technology or procedures can improve upon Natural Law, which is the same today as 5000 years ago. No technique or technology can take the place of every practitioner paying the personal price of becoming a better instrument of nature; becoming more unified and integrated with the natural laws.

- *Kind, but lax, too unspecific.*
  Patients go to a health care specialist because their bodies and their lives are out of control in some way, and they are looking, either consciously or unconsciously, for direction. Clear policy, procedures, forms, a schedule, patient report of findings, backsliding prevention procedure, progress updates, recommendations to follow — all these show and create an image of providing care aimed at successful results. When you and your staff get specific, explain 1) benefits, 2) how your procedures and equipment work to help them, and 3) how your home recommendations and treatment will help them, your patients will then quote whatever you say about this to others. The result of a <u>specific</u> program of care and education is referral.

- *Compassionate, but too eccentric.*
  Patients love a compassionate practitioner. However, if the practitioner is

too far out of the mainstream in dress, appearance, attitude and ideas, his/her patients can feel sufficiently uncomfortable to look for another practitioner. Practitioners who are less focused on promoting or preaching their particular brand of life style and who are more focused on listening to the needs of patients, don't put obstacles in the way of people coming to them.

■ *Good results, means well, but too preachy.*
Patients want good results, but not at any price. Practitioners who tend to preach "at" patients are more concerned with their good ideas, than with "relating" to the patient. Patients want to feel that their practitioners can put themselves in their shoes and understand them. More and more people want to participate and cooperate intelligently in their own care. The practitioner, for example, who works out home care instructions with the patient and elicits a willingness to work together can often gain greater success with the patient.

■ *Young, new to the profession.*
Practitioners who are young and new to the profession have to overcome the distrust of inexperience. Often young male practitioners can add a beard or moustache to appear older to help assuage anxiety over age. They also can capitalize on their youth to appeal to a younger age group and select a specialty in which they can achieve excellent results for that market. Teenagers with acne problems for example, will probably feel very comfortable going to a younger acupuncturist specializing in skin disorders because they may feel more rapport with their practitioner in understanding their dilemma. As the practitioner grows older, his or her specialties may broaden, but the young practitioner should capitalize on what he offers uniquely, and his/her age is one.

■ *Tries too hard, overly friendly.*
If practitioners are excessive in any manner with patients, it makes people both suspicious and uncomfortable. They often wonder if the practitioner is hiding something, particularly their level of competence. Practitioners who are less concerned with impressing their patients than with giving their patients room to express themselves, are the ones to whom patients will choose to return.

■ *Very quiet practitioner, doesn't say much.*
Patients must feel that the practitioner is responding to them. Often patients will come to a practitioner looking for answers, trying to understand why they have a problem, and what can be done about it, beyond

treatment. Patients want to talk about their situation to varying degrees, and they want feedback. How much discussion is wanted can be determined by asking and listening to the patient. Practitioners who make an effort to explain to patients what can be done, who ask their patients vital questions, who acknowledge what the patients are feeling, and who do touch and tell procedures are the ones with whom patients feel comfortable. The patient can trust that the practitioner can help them not just fix the condition, but correct tendencies and get to the cause.

■ *Good results, consistent policy and procedures, but lack the human warmth and touch.*
Patients want more than just technicians. They want to be supported emotionally as well as physically and mentally, to get back on the track of good health. Human warmth, rapport, compassion are priceless forms of service which provide the "extras" that make a practice unique. Practitioners who have good or excellent reputations hire staff who project this warmth, and provide it themselves. Practitioners who project not only excellence, but warmth, generate referrals.

■ *Refers out more than treats.*
Patients appreciate a practitioner's honest appraisal of what he/she can and cannot treat, in addition to being referred out appropriately. However, if referring out more than treating becomes a habit, other treating physicians and patients feel the practitioner is insecure and not making the effort to develop his/her own competencies. Practitioners become more substantial as practitioners as they expand their skill in treating patients, not conditions.

Editor's note: If we see patients only as "conditions", which we can or cannot address, we will never grow as healers. We will only be technicians.

■ *Quantity practice. Good relief results, but no long term benefit.*
A number of patients will pay low cost for relief health care. The practitioner who has a production line low cost care practice has a reputation for being cheap, not necessarily for being a quality care practitioner. Patients do look for quality and long term benefit. They are the ones who look for referrals or ads which say "total patient care" or "We treat the whole person, not just the symptom." Practitioners who deliberately plan care at whatever level they agree with patients — relief, stabilization, optimal care, and maintenance care — and do multiple appointment scheduling with planned reevaluations give their patients

opportunity to build long term health benefit through consistent goals and means.

■ *Disorganized. Inconsistent in practice, procedures, policies.*
Patients must feel that they get consistent good care each visit, **both** from the practitioner and from his staff. Patients feel they have a right to expect consistency.

Not only do they need and want consistency in their lives, they very much expect it from service people. They find it difficult to deal with people in business, including health care practices, which do not have or carry out clear policies and procedures.

The patient may get great results from treatment, but if he is having problems with your insurance clerk who fails to send the bills on time or know where the account stands, this creates considerable discomfort. If patients' calls are not returned consistently, or if they frequently wait over 15 minutes to see you, they may become irritated. If patients get good relief results, but receive no further health plan or real understanding of their problem, this is also annoying. Patients may come for a while, but may feel something is wrong without really knowing why. These patients most likely won't refer, and may eventually seek another practice in which they sense quality and consistency of policy and procedure. In sum, patients require quality not only from the practitioner, but from the staff's manner in handling phone calls, scheduling, collections, and explaining follow-through procedures.

Irritants such as those described above often happen in quantity relief care practices, or those that experience fast growth without adequate staffing to smooth out procedures and policies. Practices should plan for growth so that good, consistent patient procedures are established first. This provides a solid foundation on which to build a reputation and control expansion.

■ *Good results, but easily interruptible, distracted, preoccupied.*
For practitioners to build a reputation of credibility, patients must feel a sense of presence about the practitioner. They must feel the practitioner's attention is fully with them, not the next patient, the phone call that's

waiting, the concern about all the people in the waiting room, etc. If patients don't feel this present time awareness with them, they justify successful results in this way: "I would have gotten better anyway" or "I got results, in spite of the practitioner!" They would never refer such a practitioner.

Reputations Which Engender Negative Images:

- Bossy, self important, makes patients wait, doesn't value his patient's time or attitude
- Know-it all attitude
- Poor reputation
- Scary reputation of malpractice or negligence
- Womanizer/Hustler
- Rigid in his/her ways
- High-pressure, too rushed
- Indifferent, insensitive, doesn't hear the patient's viewpoint
- Argumentative
- Distasteful personal habits and mannerisms
- Overcontrolling

Images Which Don't Support Good Reputation-Building:

- Unspecific identity, too difficult to describe to others
- No niche in the market
- No specialties, unless it is in the individual who comes to "you" for help
- Dress code is unprofessional
- Nonprofessional attitude or mannerisms
- Outdated
- Inconsistent with appearance of self, office, location, equipment, and advertising
- Not knowing how to communicate to others about his practice
- No brochures, no advertising about the practice
- Office and location are functional only and do not convey the practitioner's interests, expertise, and love of people
- Labeled as poor man's doctor, rich-man's doctor; rules out the middle class

You can see after reading this section, how important patient and staff feedback can be in both assessing and building image and reputation.

Your Office Presentation

> ## What Message Do You Want Your Office To Convey to Your Patients?

A patient hears about your reputation from a friend, picks up an article about you, hears your front office person's tone of voice, and spends more time waiting in your reception room, consultation room, and treatment room than actually being physically present with you. Your environment sends out many messages which are representative of you. These messages are often more nonverbal than verbal and reinforced by visual perception. Presentation is the key to opening the door to your success.

Your presentation — whether it be in your advertising, the first interaction with your office by phone, where you choose to locate, how you dress, your manner with patients, your care in treatment, your office presentation — all are the primary ways you broadcast to people your concern for them. What do people sense or look for. . . ?

☐ 1. **Is the appearance of the office and practitioner inviting?**
   If your office is in a declining neighborhood or you are "too far out" in appearance, it will make any patient middle class or higher feel uncomfortable. They are the ones who can afford your services most easily. Don't cut them off. Patients like to come to an office that looks successful.

   The most inviting three office choices are: a well-kept office on a main thoroughfare, on a bus line, and one that creates no parking problem; a modern middle class neighborhood office within a newly developed area in large city (such as a shopping center); and downtown in a preferred office building with elevator service. (Preferred locations are in or near medical centers.)

☐ 2. **Are you easily accessible? Is the location convenient?**
   Or is your office difficult to get to; and once your patient gets there, is it difficult to enter? Make sure you have ample parking adjoining your office, the walkways are safe, bushes won't snag your patients

on the way in, and they aren't out of breath by climbing stairs to get to you. You want them to be alive when they enter your doors. If you're on the second floor, make sure there is an elevator. If you have frustrated patients because they can't get to you easily, you will start off your relationship with them on a sour note. Make it easy for them.

❏ 3. **Are you visible?**
Your patients have to find you easily! Do you have a sign? Is it visible? A new patient might decide not to make his appointment out of embarrassment for being late or because it was too difficult to find you. Keep your sign professional. Black silhouette is in good taste on a marquee type sign. The size of the sign should be in keeping with the size of the building. If expense is a problem, black lettering in professional good taste works well. Interior signs should be either printed or professionally lettered and framed under glass. If you practice at night, make sure the sign is well-lit and on a timer, to save expense.

❏ 4. **Is your office an environment of healing and harmony?**
What about the color scheme? Is it dull or nonexistent? Healing atmospheres are warm, friendly, bright, soothing, calming, alive, fresh. Environment can add or detract from healing and total health. The office interior should create a healing and healthful mood both in arrangement and color. Color for Healing is a good book to incorporate when creating a healthful environment. Neutral shades are good background colors—light green, light tan, ivory, with appropriate color accents to create the feeling you want. In decorating, use a store which has a free courtesy decorator to help you with colors and moods. Avoid loud colors. If you use pictures, think about their colors and subject matter. A contemporary motif is good. It's best not to use pictures with needles in them in the reception room itself. A treatment room where you demonstrate or use needles is better. Using taped healing music, sounds, colors, crystals, aquariums, plants, and artistic touches such as sculptures can maximize an atmosphere of healing in your practice. Patients want to be able to feel comfortable and relaxed in a healing office. Ask yourself, "What can I do to create a healing environment for my patients?"

❏ 5. **Is the office neat and clean?**
You may be so dedicated you don't see the forest for the trees, or the dirt all around you. You don't want your patients to feel embarrassed to refer another patient to an office because it wasn't clean. Hire a

professional cleaner on a regular basis for your office upkeep. Ask your office personnel to keep an eye on the office throughout the day. The treatment table paper must be changed, the bathrooms must be fresh, the desks and tables neat, and the carpets spot-cleaned as needed.

☐ **6. Is the office well-organized?**
People associate a cluttered office with a cluttered mind. Patients expect you, your office, and your staff to be organized and their paperwork and condition handled in a timely, efficient, and caring way. Patients ask themselves, "Do I want to be treated by a practitioner or staff who appear to be scattered?"

☐ **7. Is the office well-lit?**
Does the office feel and look dingy? Do the walls look like they were painted over a year ago, or if they were painted, does it look sterile? Does natural daylight stream through the windows? If so, you had better light and paint your office. Lighting should be indirect. Certain fluorescent tubes are all right, using a combination of cool-white and daylight tubes alternately in each fixture. Some florescent lighting creates headaches. Utilize as much natural sunlight as possible. Patients don't want to come to a dingy office. They want to see a brighter day, and feel lighter!

☐ **8. Is the office soundproof?**
Patients want to have the feeling of privacy. They don't want to overhear what happens in the room next door, and they certainly don't want other people to hear confidential information about themselves. You don't want your patient to withhold important information regarding their health or stifle their expression with you. If they can't confide, they will quit. Soundboard, carpeting, acoustical tile, certain partitions, solid core doors, various insulating materials can all be used. If you can't remodel your present office, it would be wise to move.

☐ **9. Does your office smell fresh?**
Or does it have an odor? Smells can attract or repel your patients. Make sure the rooms have proper ventilation or air purifiers, and are sprayed with room deodorants. Two main considerations: One, while moxa may contribute to healing, its smell can be strong and offensive to some people. You want to prevent the odor from infiltrating the hallway or neighboring offices. You might be asked to leave the building. This could cause unnecessary expense. You should not let moxa's smell upset people in your office, either. Two: You need to

take measures to insure your patients health once they enter your office. Consider a "No Smoking" policy and sign in your office. Ask yourself," "Does my office smell inviting enough for my patients? Would they invite their friends and family to come?"

☐10. **Is your office up-to-date and your equipment well cared for? Does your office look like it belongs in present time?**
Or, is the furniture outdated, or worn? Do the walls look dingy? Are the magazines in the office outdated? Your furniture should be of professional design, not living room variety. Tables should match or be in harmony with the entire color scheme. Use mirrors in the dressing/ treatment room. Desk tops can be covered with glass to give a finished appearance. Your equipment may not be the latest model, but if it is polished, clean, and modern looking, it will appear more up-to-date. Keep current reading magazines in your front office on both health related and general human interest.

Patients may think that if you don't care to update your office, you may not care enough to update your equipment, or that you fail to keep abreast of the latest advances in the medical field. If you can't see as far as your front office, they may well wonder how far *you can* see.

☐11. **Does your office easily accommodate your patients, their friends and family?**
Or is the office too busy, too cramped, or too empty? Patients don't like to feel insignificant, claustrophobic, or removed. If your office has any of the above symptoms, they can be remedied by 1) correct scheduling of patients so that there is a moderate flow of patients through the office at any one time and 2) an appropriate amount of furniture, space, interest, as well as time, to accommodate your patients. Ask yourself, "Can I accommodate my patients, their friends, and families comfortably?"

☐12. **Does your office motivate others to learn more about their health and about you?**
Does it contribute to their trust in you and hope for themselves? I recently saw a door mat in front of a health office which said, "Take a step to your health." Then as I walked through the door, my gaze immediately lit upon a sign which said, "The purpose of our clinic is to support as many people as possible in their quest for health, and to educate them about _____ (acupuncture, ibid.) so they may, in turn, educate others." Below it there was a long display rack well filled with pamphlets written for the patient (stamped with the

practitioners name, address and phone), each on a different condition and how _____ (substitute "acupuncture") treats the condition. On the top of the rack was a card holder which said, "If you have a condition for which you need assistance, I would be pleased to meet with you for a courtesy consultation. Please ask the receptionist to arrange a time. If you have a friend who might benefit from these pamphlets, please take what you need to share". A friend, who was waiting for a patient, walked over and chose two pamphlets, and began reading. She leaned over to me and said, "You know I didn't know acupuncture treated _____. I think I will make an appointment." It was a colorful office alive with a waterfall, plants, an interesting blend of pictures, a big round table in the middle of the room with human interest magazines, health magazines, and a testimonial book, in which patients had written notes and letters about their change in health and how they had been helped. There were even before and after pictures in the book. What a difference in their expression. I watched another person flip through the book and smile thoughtfully. I wondered how much impact this book and the atmosphere had on this practitioner's credibility and the patient's hope for healing.

☐13. **Ask yourself, "Does this office increase the patient's confidence in me?"**
All of actions described above are conveyed by the environment you create, and add to the patient's confidence in the practitioner. Another important point is to display your diplomas. They should be nicely, even beautifully, framed on the wall in the consultation room and treatment room, demonstrating that you are not only qualified, but up-to-date in the latest procedures.

SUCCESSFUL offices are inclusive, accessible, and visible; inspiring and harmonious; organized; bright, fresh, and inviting; comfortable and accommodating; up-to-date and motivating. These are attributes that create a credible image. They inspire confidence in the acupuncturist, and furthermore, *display* the attitudes of health and well-being.

How to Create Your Image with Your Office

In the previous section we considered the importance of color, plants, smells, light, sound, cleanliness, being up to date, space, and educational materials in regard to healing and patient comfort. Here are some specific ways you can build your practice and practitioner image:

Image: **Competence.** Your diplomas, continuing education classes taken, framed articles you have written and submitted to newspapers with pictures of you in a professional setting.

Image: **Healthy, warm human being.** Other pictures and articles about you which tell them something about your personality, your self-image, your health awareness.

Image: **Excellence and dedication.** Recognition awards or trophies for civic service, for hospital service with children, for rehabilitation work with addictive patients, for excellence in any field from sports to flower arranging.

Image: **Successful healer.** Testimonials by patients with before and after photos placed in a photo album in your office. Newspaper articles with testimonials and pictures of patients who have gotten good results.

Image: **Showing that you care.** Special touches around your office such as tea and water in the waiting room for patients, flowers in the reception room, spotlessly clean and painted bathroom with a simple, beautiful, or funny framed picture.

Image: **Your love of people.** Include pictures, magazines, and articles in your office that tell people who and what you love: Have a few interesting magazines in your reception room which have human interest stories in them: Life Magazine, Sports Illustrated, etc.

Image: **Acupuncture as a respected profession.** Place the *American Journal of Acupuncture* and other respected acupuncture magazines, journals and articles in a notebook in your reception room, which emphasize articles about acupuncture today--it's benefits and aids, and scientific backing.

Image: **Your speciality in particular conditions or type of practice.** If you want to build a children's practice, frame children's pictures, or have books and playthings in a kiddy corner for them. If you want people to know you are interested in developing your practice around those involved in sports, include sports magazines, sports trophies, articles of interest to sports patients, such as brochures for sports injuries. If you focus on skin rejuvenation and beauty, rejuvenate your office with aesthetic skin tone colors, focus on including magazines on beauty and health, brochures on how acupuncture rejuvenates, and add aesthetic pictures which make people reflect the impression they want to have.

Image: **Welcoming of more patients.** Include the "We Love Referrals" pamphlet in your waiting room. Have enough comfortable chairs so your patients can bring their friends and families.

Image: **Modern and progressive.** Have everything up to date: a well organized health care classroom, videos, audiotapes, magazines in your reception room such as *Prevention Magazine, East West Journal,* scientific journals, sports magazines (if this is your emphasis), *Life,* brochure racks and brochures with your name and phone number stamped on them, which keep people informed of ways to function healthier in today's world.

*   *   *   *

The section on "Reaching Your Patients," "Creating Reputation and Image," and the later section on "Patient Visit Procedure" provide the *foundation* and for your reputation and marketing approach. <u>Volume IV, Patient Communication, Public Relations and Marketing</u> provide more of the examples and specifics.

FINANCIAL PLANNING AND MANAGEMENT

Preparing a Financial Foundation

Look at financially planning as an adventure in both charted and unchartered territory. Your job as the adventurer is to look at all the angles and find the best way to navigate through the waters towards your goal.

One of your tools to use is mathematics. Now math is essential for the operations of your practice and an important part of your practice financial planning. Using it will mean the difference between sailing or sinking. As an adventurer you might have a tendency, feeling the surge of the adventure, to just plunge in and trust everything will take care of itself in time. However, if you have a tendency to want to skip over the mathematical planning, hold the ship. Otherwise, you will find yourself constantly adrift and unable to control your practice financially. Financial planning is one area that intuitive thinking isn't geared to do. Financial planning is left brain work. If you can't bring yourself to do it, get help from a mentor who has successful experience in financial planning a practice.

Another factor to keep in mind. Financial planning can enhance your relationship with others, or on the other hand, it can ruin it. In order to get loans, even from relatives, others appreciate your willingness to be clear with them . Everyone wants you to do well-- your mother, your husband or wife, your banker, both creditors and friends. But no one wants you to do what you do at their mental, physical, or emotional expense. Even if they have all the money in the world, and giving it away for them is like water falling off a duck's back, you wouldn't want poor financial planning to disturb your relationship with them. It's often easier to get more funds up front than to have to go back later and ask for more. Coming up short creates short levels of trust in their mental, emotional, and physical bank account. People lend to you because they have faith in you. Give yourself and them all the reason in the world to make that loan good by putting in your best planning and implementing it. You will find out soon enough if the plan is workable. If parts don't work, be flexible and adjust it.

"What if you can't make good," you think. Does this mean that you must be paralyzed by the fear of making financial mistakes? Paralysis does happen, believe me. However, remind yourself that you are human and you will make mistakes. I don't know of any truly successful men and women who have not made mistakes in financial planning.

If financial planning is uncomfortable for you, and I assure you, it is uncomfortable for almost everyone, start by remembering why you are doing it. Then consider your objectives, resources, and what kind of outcome you want to see. You want your practice to succeed, and no one wants to feel that their efforts are in vain. Then get out your #2 pencils, extra paper, your eraser, a box of kleenex, and start filling in your financial figures in this estimating section. As you fill in your figures, keep your goals in mind.

Use your insight and strategic planning as you work with your figures and consider the financial planning factors appropriate for your state of practice. (See Financial Planning Goals by Stages of Practice", next section).

1. Identify and keep your financial goals in mind.
2. Choose your most important goal and objective and proceed with that single goal in mind.
3. Rearrange your assets in various ways to test what brings you closer to your goal.
4. Rearrange your liabilities in various ways to test what brings you closer to your goal.
5 Try multiple rearrangements to see if any of the combinations are better than a single move.
6. Review the impact of the various rearrangements to see which, if any achieve multiple goals.
7. Then have your financial plan reviewed by a professional.

Before you present your figures to a banker or anyone else for a loan, ask someone you trust for some referrals and interview those who will be on your financial management team. Then have one of them review your figures--someone like an accountant, financial planner, or community service representative from an organization such as the Service Corp of Retired Executives (SCORE).

Keep in mind that a successful financial objective is to create the means to establish the proper relation of expenses to income production, stable cash flow, and make a profit.

Financial Planning Goals by Stages of Practice

Pre-Start Up Stage

Goals:

- To save funds for initial opening.

- To plan strategically your income and expenses

- To plan financial impact and outside funding.

- To set your financial plan in place and apply for funds.

- To do accurate set up, income, cost, and monthly expenses projections.

- To schedule realistic cash flow figures, dates of large amounts of payments due.

- To set income strategy (use demographic and psychographic research on target patients for specialty as well as location; and procedures.

- To plan not only your financial funding, but tax strategy, who will handle accounting management, billing procedure, and legal structure.

- To set your financial management team in place - banker, lawyer, accountant, free professional services advice, consultant.

- To write up list of fees, services, fee incentives and discounts to spur cash flow, and guidelines for implementing fees.

- To setup type of financial system.

- To write or adapt financial policy to use.

- To determine financial management control forms to use (forms in *Big Forms Packet* and the *Insurance Forms Packet*).

- To arrange for loan or leasing for practice purchases to purchase furnishings, equipment and supplies.

- To setup bookkeeping system, merchant mastercard visa, and billing system.

- To setup insurance billing forms, procedures.

- To learn about and decide on collection procedure, scheduling.

- To set health care planning, forms, and follow-through procedures in place.

- To set referral building plan in place.

- To hire motivated and dedicated part time staff.

- To set marketing methods and costs in place with effective marketing and advertising.

- To set appropriate rental and lease agreements in force, fees and agreements for renters in your space.

- To arrange for loan or leasing for practice purchases.

- To purchase furnishings, equipment and supplies.

Start-up phase to stabilization:

Goal: to obtain new patients and referrals.

Focus: to give quality care and educate people to a "preference" for acupuncture care.

How: Promote quality care. Give extra time and attention, recommendations, directions, supportive health care products, etc.

How: (See marketing chapter and marketing plan for examples, plus *Volume IV*. When you have ten patients, initiate a required health care class where patients bring at least one support person.)

Goal: To increase volume in proportion to consistent quality service.

How: (Don't increase volume faster than you can give good service). Use your marketing and referral building plan.

Goal: To establish cash flow balance.

How: Redefine turnover rate and adjust marketing and referral procedure accordingly. Monitor your financial policy --what works and what doesn't. (Use management control forms to help you with this.)

Goal: To establish your preferred patient type(s) and educated health care planning system.

How: Market to your specialty group, and bring up your specialty with patients. Display pamphlets on your specialty. Advertise your specialty. Establish in an area where your specialty is preferred. Set your office theme around your specialty.

How: Educate your patients beyond relief care. Do multiple appointment scheduling with reevaluation.

How: Establish your networking referral base around your specialty.

Goal: Referrals from other practitioners.

How: Free time to network with other practitioners by delegating front office work and paperwork. (See marketing section).

Goal: To keep within your budget; to make sure your initial costs carry you through the first 18 months of practice.

How: Pay attention to the factors on the expense and income control list.

Goal: To iron out trouble spots in procedure.

How: See practice pitfalls, as well as staff management section. Read **Volume II** for background.

Goal: Follow-through care without patient financial burden or creating cash flow crunch for you.

How: Don't give up until you find a bank to give you a merchant mastercard / visa account. Promote credit cards as primary patient payment option.

Stabilization :

Goal in itself.
How: Focus on consistency in the quality of your services and monitor cash flow with management control forms.

Stabilization to growth phase:

Goal in itself. (Look at the direction you want growth to take, patient type, quality of care, etc.)

How: Activate marketing plan to increase specific type of new patient volume. Add new productive procedures one at a time. Include liberalized insurance policy and credit procedures.

Plateau phase:

Goal: Enjoy the level off or reevaluate approach.

How: Reevaluate pitfalls section on slowdown growth. Adapt to create what you want.

Growth phase to expansion phase:	**Goal in itself:** (Look at quality care/volume/income ratio and pitfalls to set more specific goals)
	How: Put greater profits into the business to expand services, health care products, modalities. Expand health care classes. Add staff to increase and handle the increase of consistent quality patient service, volume, and income. Enhance facilities.
Expansion phase:	**Goal in itself.** (Look at benefits and pitfalls.)
	How: Take a directorship role with associates and colleagues under you. Add another office to expand services further. Sell the practice. Reinvest the funds in long term income-producing or tax saving investments and start or buy another.
Level off phase:	**Goal in itself.** (Look at benefits future retirement.)
	How: Reduce in practice time. Sell the practice. Take a directorship role with very little treating. Continue by providing quality in-depth services and less quantity services. Hire others to run the practice. Phase out everything but teaching. Write a book; Retire from the profession completely. Explore another aspect of life.

Practice Income Picture

The following presentation is to give you a visual idea of what particular income sources financial affect your practice. It is important to visualize both inflow -- and outflow -- so you can approach your practice realistically.

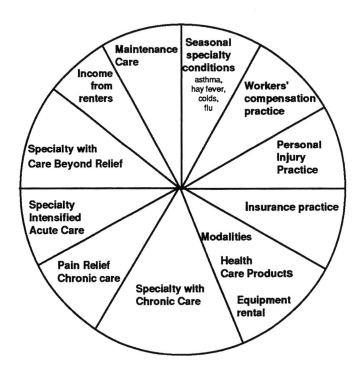

Specialty: _____
Specialty: _____
Seasonal specialty: _____

Predominate patient type: (conditions, ages, sex, socio-economic background) _____
_____
_____
Acute care balance (%):_____
Chronic care balance (%) _____

Practitioner referrals of % acute care: _____
Practitioner referrals of % chronic care:____

Patient referrals of % acute care: ____
Patient referrals of % chronic care: ____

% Income from acupuncture   ____

% Income from consultations   ____
% Income from modalities   ____
% Income from equipment rental   ____
% Income from health care products   ____

Current gross monthly income:
% Income from cash, mastercard/visa ____
% Income from insurance practice   ____
% Income from workers' compensation____
% Income from litigation/personal injury
____
% Income from payment plans   ____
% Past due 60,75,90 days pt. income   ____
                                       ____
                                       ____
% monthly Collection of gross income ____
% Income from other sources
        professiional and/or renters   ____
        loans   ____
        savings   ____
        other _____   ____

Income Generating Factors

One major reasons practitioners have trouble either creating or building their practice is the frustration at not being able to see how their mental, emotional, physical, and financial decisions relate to their patient growth, type of practice, or procedures; to the feeling tone of the practice; to their personal or practice's reputation and image; or to their cash flow or income level. This section should give you greater insight into these relationships.

Your income is affected by how you establish fees, the type of services, procedures, and products you use in your niche and locale; and importantly, your manner of delivery. Your income will be greatly influenced by the balance between acute and chronic care in your practice. Your willingness to set moral and realistic income patterns will also be influenced by a sense of moral and financial obligation to meet your expenses and financial goals. The below factors greatly influence the basis for setting-up your fees, services and products.

1. The **value you set** on the services and products you offer.
    Most practitioners consider their time, skill, and knowledge, level of complexity, diagnosis, and type of treatment involved for their services when setting their fees. Their fee is a reflection of their self-worth, training, expertise, as well as time and type of care.

    The value practitioners set reflect the quality of service -- both desirable and required for the type of patients they serve.

    The value set reflects the results a practitioner achieves with those services, and what a patient would have to pay elsewhere for to achieve like results within the whole medical marketplace. This speaks for the practitioner's experience. Generally, established practitioners have built a history of success and they feel justified in charging accordingly.

    A practitioner must still keep perspective and look at "usual, customary, and reasonable" fees which other practitioners charge in the market place. However, remember: the charges of other doctors are based on what *they* see their worth as. The value set on services ultimately comes down to one's own sense of value.

Most successful practitioners tend to rank success of results first in setting fees, with skill, and expertise next; then complexity, diagnosis, with time last. Practice consultant Robert Levoy notes an interesting phenomenon often occurs with fee raising: a raise in fees = better service = exuberant practitioner = enthusiastic patients = greater income = office improvements = better equipment and decor = more referrals = greater success. It seems to be a time honored economic law: "Success begets success."

2. **Value others place on your fees.**

   Patients feel increased or higher fees are justified in almost all cases for good results, extra services, extra time, recommendations, empathy, understanding, and compassion. How much faith the assistant has in you, how confident, sensitive, and creative she is in asking for fees, will determine how successful your fee is. If your front office assistant can't convey your value in fee collection or promotion, get an assistant who can. General insurance companies tend to rank payment of fees based on usual, customary and reasonable charges within the medical profession for "specific diagnosis." Setting successful fees will be discussed later.

3. **Insurance practice** (in states and countries where it is legal.)

   Certain economic realities, such as income from insurance payment ensures that care will be remunerated for the practitioner's services without burden to the patient. Income from this source allows greater follow-through care. It generally provides greater receivable income because many patients would need to stop patient care, had it not been for insurance coverage. Insurance payment can provide the practitioner with that added justification to purchase equipment which not only adds to patient health, but will be paid for more quickly because that specific equipment use is covered by patient insurance. It behooves the practitioner, in states where acupuncture is covered by insurance, to provide for insurance handling within his practice so that income from insurance payment is ensured.

   Preparation to handle income from insurance should occur at the beginning of practice. This means getting your insurance paperwork setup, your collection and follow-up procedure set. At the beginning, you may need to accept payment in full upon service (cash, check, or mastercard/visa) and give the patient a superbill for reimbursement. In the growth phase, you are freer to liberalize your financial policy and take "assignment of insurance benefits" with patient payment of the deductible only upon service.

4. **Patient type (statistics by payment method, turnover, and cash flow)**

From a business perspective, predominately acute care practices have a high turnover rate. Predominately chronic care practices have a low turnover rate with stability. Workers' compensation and insurance paying cases provide stable accounts receivables, but not necessarily stable cash flow. Cash or mastercard/visa paying patients and patients with insurance who pay at the time of service and are reimbursed by insurance, provide the greatest cash flow and stabilize a practice. Most of your stable practices are predominately chronic care. Set your ledger cards up as suggested in *Volume II* under "Office Procedure for Billing: Choosing your billing system. "Then use the "Management Control Form #3" in the *Big Forms Packet* to see what your statistics area. This is important! Whatever balance you build into your practice, you must compensate by your socioeconomic location, your fee level, the way your inspire referrals, who you ask to refer, and what kind of advertising you will do.

5. **The type of practice, socioeconomic area, and specialty you serve.**

You may have explored some specialty areas which you could promote to potential patients. See if you can discern the percentages (listed on the income wheel page) which you are anticipating or experiencing in your practice. Is this what is in your highest interest from the standpoint of practice stability?

Consider the demographics and psychographics carefully in the area in which you want to practice. There may be parts of the population in the area in which you want to practice which are not being reached. Your Department of Health will have the demographics and psychographics in your area for particular health conditions. You may be surprised at untapped parts of the population who could use your services if you would market directly to them. It is essential to 1) find the markets which will stabilize your practice income as well as 2) provide a valuable service to others.

If you are already in practice, you should have some idea of the kind of patients which your way of practicing tends to attract. These patients have demographic and psychographic qualities to them, and have some interesting similarities, whether it be socioeconomic background, predominately similar conditions, age bracket, ethnic background, predominately relief care, predominately acute care, high, medium, or low cash payers, high, medium, or low percentage of insurance patients, etc., and they often refer other people of like kind. Thus, your practice takes a particular appearance. The following are four scenarios to show how type of practice, socioeconomic area, and specialty affect the difference in fee bases and income generation.

Practitioner A 1) doesn't specialize, 2) charges a flat rate for his time, 3) offers a basic-treatment-only-type-of-practice, 4) no recommendations, education, or office enhancement, and 5) pays rent in a low income neighborhood with 6) high acupuncture acceptance. He is more likely to develop:

1. A quantity-type-of-practice
2   High patient volume
3. Low fees typical of what patients can pay in the neighborhood

Practitioner B is an acupuncturist, located in a 1) middle class area 2) medical complex, 3) who specializes in screening blood pressure and regulating circulatory problems. He will probably have:

1. A mix of patients from a variety of socioeconomic backgrounds
2. Predominately elderly on insurance and Medicare
3. Cases would range from simple to complex and require blood work, case conferences with other physicians, and at times sophisticated diagnostic equipment, or equipment sharing. He would take into consideration his patient base, the fact that his is:
4. A Chronic care practice
5. Low turnover
6. Mid range standard fees in the medical profession for blood pressure, cardiac checks, and maintenance care
7. Products might include nutritional supplements, herbs, cushions, mag netic items, (exception, perhaps pacemakers patients), relaxation tapes

Practitioner C is 1) family practice oriented 2) in a middle class neighborhood, 3) around families and children, 4) promotes preventative health care 5) education, and 6) maintenance care.

1. Turnover is moderate
2. Prices will probably reflect moderate pricing for the medical field
3. Additional moderately priced products oriented towards health mainte nance will add income to this type of practice

Practitioner D is 1)a skin rejuvenation and face-lifts specialist 2) paying rent in a middle to higher class neighborhood. His practice is more oriented toward 3) higher socioeconomic patients, predominantly female, who are used to 4) paying surgical prices for like services. A successful practice with this specialty and neighborhood is likely to be:

1. A high turnover practice
2. Personal care practice with extra time, education, equipment, attention to office beauty enhancers, and services oriented towards quality individualized attention
3. The fees would be higher because of the type of specialization, as well as to offset a lower volume of patients
4. Beauty creams, magnetic jewelry, support cushions would probably be offered at higher prices and would naturally be offered with this type of practice with increased income

Socioeconomic level of the neighborhood affects patient perception of the fee. Type of specialty has a reputation for higher or lower fees and services, as well as more to less expensive equipment and products. Certain specialties require more aesthetic atmospheres than others, greater expenses to maintain and higher fees. Quantity practices will vary in fee base success according to which class of neighborhood they are in. Specialty can affect the speed of patient turnover in a practice, so marketing, advertising, and referral building dialogue has to balance this. Products which enhance services and home recommendations up the income of all niches of practices.

* **Note:** For our purposes here, we are discussing product sales from the standpoint of expanding **needed** services with the potential for expanded income. We are not purporting recommendations of products and services based on the pocketbook to patients.

6. **Income generators are any procedure, fee, or service you initiate or add which passes the tests of producing 1) cooperation, 2) reputation 3) results, 4) follow-through care 5) lifelong relationship and 6) referrals.**

These are effective overall for your practice and are patient motivators which inspire patients to want and have better health and produce patient commitment and enthusiasm. These are procedures which increase a practice without resulting in hassles or stress and make you feel like you accomplished something by the end of the day.

The following procedures and the way you carry them out can *stabilize patient care and practice income simultaneously:* the treatment and health care planning system, written recommendations, schedule, and directions for home care, multiple appointment scheduling with immediate report of findings and progress reevaluation visit, recalls and backsliding prevention and procedures.

These procedures also include the following procedures which **contribute to patient growth and growth of income**: understanding, caring, and courteous attitude, explanation of various benefits, explanation of short and long term results, touch and tell procedures, reinforcing progress, consultation with other current physicians, the way you use audiovisual aids, the way you use patient fill-in progress reports, patient reevaluations and feedback, acupuncture orientation and health care classes, an on time practice, smooth payment and scheduling procedure, thank you letters, liberalized insurance policies, family plans, wellness plans, clear office and financial procedures, efficient insurance billing system, current equipment which doesn't increase overhead excessively, good office appearance, fresh advertising directed toward specialty or niche, asking for referrals, educating with pamphlets.

7. **Harmonizing both moral and financial goals and obligations.**
    As a healer, a practitioner turns away no one in need, and recommends care based on the patient's need and what will assist him to greatest health. A practitioner separates financial considerations from treatment recommendations. He is ethical in his approach. As a businessman, a practitioners must be equally objective in taking the healthiest approach to income planning, building stability, growth and expansion.

    Your fees, as well as the type of services, and products you offer are the reasonable standard not only to meet patient health care goals, but to meet your financial goals and obligations—paying your business bills, your employees, your taxes, your living expenses, expanding your business, and making a profit. Fees, services and products must be decided upon carefully in order to meet your goals.

    In any case you must substantially more than offset your expenses, and more than just consider fees, adding more products or types of services, location, your specialty, the type of practice balance between acute care and chronic care, marketing and enthusiastic referring patients. You must notice the difference between your "Actual and Projected Income and Expenses" and balance your income with "Where Much of an Office Fee Goes." (These pages are in *Volume I*)

    Self-worth, practicality, and altruism, must be weighed carefully, as well as the various kind of "extras" in service, supplies and equipment you offer. These elements, for example, will all dramatically affect fee setting, time use, your choice of socioeconomic area impacts, your willingness to carry out appropriate financial policies, and generate revenues.

Keep your moral, financial goals, your business goals, and your marketing goals and obligations in sight and keep them in proper perspective. To stay in business, you must give full value for what you charge your patients, for patient service is your life-blood. To stay in business you must profit by 1) finding ways to charge fair fees , 2) increase fees as needed at the minimum with inflation, 3) find other ways of increasing income, such as renting out and investing, 4) increase popular and desirable services and products, and 5) inspire new patients and referrals; To grow, you must neither overcharge or undervalue your fees, services and products; for, you want to have right means to fulfill your goals and dreams both professionally and personally.

Income Planning and Management

Focus your mind on realizing those practice areas and procedures addressed in the last section which 1) set your practice on a firm foundation and 2) stabilize your income most quickly. This can create less stress in your experience and greater satisfaction. It will also allow your practice to develop in a manner more supportive of you -- and everyone around you. The following points will assist you in your planning and income management process.

1. **Give more than expected.**
   The best guarantee of increased income is to give more than expected to patients, educate them about what you do, and inspire them to refer.

2. **Identify your specialties, patient types, turnover, and volume,** then your referral and marketing approaches can assist your practice to achieve not only balanced growth, but what your income trends will be.

3. **Assess financial policies, demographics and psychographics for cash flow:**
   Your demographic and psychographic patient / location study, the laws of your state, and the ability of patients to get acupuncture coverage from their insurance companies will give you information to formulate what kind of financial policy you will set up which will stimulate greater income through the practice without upsetting cash flow. Remember that high accounts receivable do not equal cash in hand to pay your expenses. How liberal you can be on payment plans or insurance assignment of benefits will depend on if you are a new practice dependent on high cash flow or whether you have a stable enough patient base already which

allows you to modify and liberalize your extension of credit. Liberalize your policy as soon as you have stable cash flow.

4. **Set appropriate fees, and aim to meet financial goals.**
   Be aware that being successful in business means setting your goals high enough and your fees at an appropriate rate to not only cover your operating costs and pay you a draw, but yield you a profit at the end of the year.

   Use the breakeven and profit formula. Your business must make a profit if it is to continue year after year and pay back the money you have invested in it. After your initial capital investment, the major source of money is your services and any additional adjuncts with your services. What dollar volume of business do you expect to do in the next 6 months? 12 months? Keep this is perspective.

5. **Charge for different levels of service and by type of diagnosis.**

6. **Promote to specific markets which provide stable financial income base.**
   Primarily low turnover chronic care conditions, maintenance care patients.

7. **Promote to specific markets which provide growth of income base.**
   Examples: workers' compensation and insurance cases. These provide stable accounts receivables, but not necessarily stable cash flow. You can establish your general insurance policy to promote cash flow, however. Focus on government employees and self-insured employer based companies in states and countries which cover acupuncture care.

8. **Address seasonal conditions.**
   Slump seasons may occur because people tend to focus their cash at certain times of the year and tend to hold onto it at other times. This often happens just prior to Christmas time and around tax season. Certain seasons people go away on vacation. However, these seasons are prime seasons for addressing certain kinds of conditions. Note the conditions which occur during these times, i.e. colds, flu, hay fever, etc. These conditions are "more priority" health care conditions during this time. For people to experience a preference for your services during this time, you must let people know specifically how you can serve them best during this time. Focus benefits in your advertising and communications with patients just before and during seasonal outbreaks. A number of practitioners schedule their patients for preventative care and send them reminder cards prior to the season.

9. **Health care planning and backsliding prevention and procedures listed earlier.**

    Offering stable and optimal health care planning = patient satisfaction, greater lasting wellness, enthusiasm, loyalty, referrals = stable and optimal growth, steady predictable income, financial stability, and good will.

    If a practitioner does not do health care planning beyond symptom relief, his patients experience unstable health. A practitioner's income level often simultaneously experiences instability. How does this happen? Patients who are not made aware of follow-through care for health stability come in for care erratically. There is never truly a sense of lasting satisfaction, and hence lower referrals. While health care planning should **never** be done based on the pocket book, it is important to be aware that lack of health care planning most often means lower patient satisfaction, lower referrals, unplanned growth, and practice instability of volume and income.

10. **Add health care products which turnover quickly.**

    Standard mark up is 50-100%. Check with the health product wholesaler for standard mark up regarding their products.
    (See worksheet for product sales in this volume)

11. **Teach classes or give presentations in specialty field for additional income and patient referrals.**

    See marketing section.

12. **Proper implementation of fees.**

    Use the acupuncturist's fee slips, and post a fee schedule at the front desk so that consistent presentation of fees to the patient does occur.

13. **Accurate and up-to-date recording.**

    Often times practitioners do not record additional time charges or extra modalities given the patient, or the assistant misses recording charges. Use the acupuncturist's fee slips (in Volume II) and fill it out accurately. This tends to prevent under and overcharging. Record **all** charges. If you don't charge for additional time or modalities, *record* N/C (no charge) on your fee slip. This at least lets patients know you gave "extra" which adds to their appreciation, as well as enthusiasm for your practice.

14. **Manner used on the telephone initially with patients regarding fees, in over the counter collections, and in scheduling.**

    People are sensitive to the tone of service and they need to know what to expect. Your initial communication with patients should clearly communicate what services you cover, the amount of time of service and the quality of services provided for the cost. If you cannot give exact cost figures, do communcate a range of cost and when and how the fee is payable. Specific and clear itemization of fees, and concern for follow-through care, add to your reputation and increased volume. If they sense this is missing, you lose patients and income.

15. Have a collection policy and procedure.
This should be built in at the same time you make your financial policy. (**Volume II** is specific on this. Note the format in this volume for creating your yown collection policy.)

16. Proper billing procedures.
Billing should be done on a specific schedule 1-2 times monthly at the same time every month. This is vital to keep cash flow moving. Insurance should be keep current and behind no more than 3 days. All services should be billed, even if no charge is written after the services. This can at least add value to patient rapport. Accurate billing saves time, energy, and money.

17. Follow-through on collections from an accounts receivable aging analysis.
A planned follow-through reminder system to late payers, and calls to insurance patients who can contact their companies at the 45 day point will increase cash flow and volume of income. Lack of timely follow-through means dead accounts receivables. Accounts receivable can be three times gross plus ten percent without being abnormal. A higher accounts receivable ratio than this indicates an out of balance practice and/or poor financial policies, or collection procedure.

18. Steady increase of new patients and services performed.
(See section "What Makes Your Practice Grow ")

19. Employee teamwork, which is productive and builds good morale.
Patients need to feel that they got full value. They can pick this up from both you, your employee, and your office presentation. Patient success is largely managing their experience so they feel good about you. Patient care omissions cause drop-outs and switching. If staff is unmotivated or negative, even though your service professionally is excellent, you can lose patients. Inspiring your staff's loyalty, enthusiasm, and managing the clarity of procedure is also controlling and managing your income.

20. Rental space income.

Taking on other professionals as renters in your space can help cash flow until your practice expands into the need for greater space. If you sublet, make sure your lease contract states you can do this.

If you have professionals rent in your space, either part-time or full time, make sure your contracts are specific for the cost of services which you provide. If there is a pro rata share of expenses, have your bookkeeper keep on top of these, so that revenues are not lost. These payments should come in on a timely basis to keep your cash flow positive.

21. Monitor your income and cash flow.

The purpose of your financial control system (statistics) is to give you current facts with an emphasis on finding the trouble spots. Use practice management controls forms in the *Big Forms Packet*. Assess where most of your income is being generated and with *what* services. (Note section on how to monitor your practice.)

The financial control system which you set up should give you information on the volume number of patients, number of new patients, dollar amount of your services, which services produce what dollar amount, where your accounts receivables are tied up, your profit, and profit and loss relationship.

22. Invest your income to increase your yield, and tax plan wisely to take advantage of legitimate savings.

See a professional financial planner and tax planner to discuss investments which will bring greater returns and savings.

23. Create your own wheel of specialties.

Dr. Fernandez points out for every condition you turn from a weak point to your strong point it potentially increases your practice growth (ibid. as well as income) by 25%.What conditions or specialties will you develop and promote?

Use the income wheel at the start of this section or create your own. If you are new in practice, from where are you planning your income? From where does the majority of your income come if you are presently in practice? How might you adjust the direction of your income?

Where Much of an Office Fee Goes

Acupuncture education
Acupuncture school loans
Postgraduate acupuncture courses

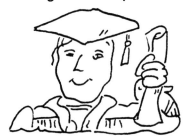

Employees' pay and benefits
Salaries
Vacations and sick pay
Medical Insurance
Life Insurance
Retirement Fund
Uniform allowances
Education allowances

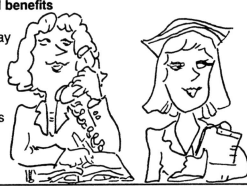

Office occupancy and maintenance
Rent or mortgage payments
Decorating
Janitorial services

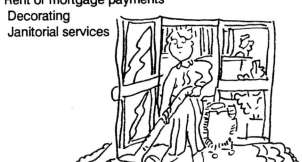

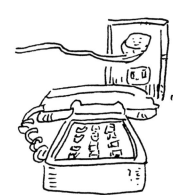
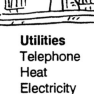

Utilities
Telephone
Heat
Electricity
Water

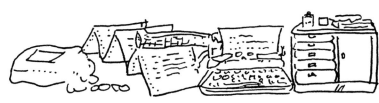

Supplies and equipment
Herbs, health products
Diagnostic and treatment equipment
Laboratory supplies
Equipment maintenance contracts
Furniture

Stationery and forms
Postage
Music
Magazines and book
Linen

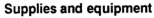

Outside Services
Legal	Laundry
Accounting	Laboratory
Telephone	Messenger
answering	Advertising & Marketing

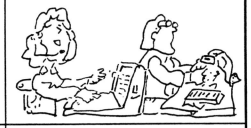

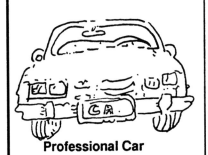

Professional Car
Operating costs
Depreciation
Licenses

Insurance
Professional liability
General liability
Property
Automobile
Workers' compensation
Bonding

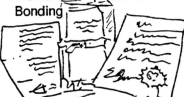

Federal, state and local taxes
Income
Real estate
Social security
Payroll
Sales

Expense Planning and Management

1. **Expenses for location and office presentation must be weighed , as well as type of patient attraction, volume, income, and cash flow.**

   (Do demographic and psychographic surveys on patient/location). For your specialty, will the expense you pay for location be the best situation to attract higher patient volume and income?

   Consider the section on advantages and disadvantages of office space. If it is legal in the area you want to practice, start off your practice in a well cared for home-professional appearing office combination, or gain experience as an associate where you don't have the large risk of financial outlay. Lease in an area that you can afford—where your referral network with both practitioners and patients indicates strength.

   A number of practitioners rent office space 2-3 days a week and increase rental space as they get busier. The disadvantage is that they don't have the degree of front office staff loyalty and training to promote them.

   Make sure the lease and utility agreement is equitable and favorable now and for the future.

   If it's more advantageous to you to lease a bigger space and rent out space to practitioners, this will bring you income until you can afford to expand into those rooms.

2. **Outlay capital in relationship to return for your investment.**
   Consider your outlay of large capital items carefully before you purchase or lease them, particularly your monthly obligation and the amount of return for your investment. Time your purchases with your growth. Use the sheets in the "Estimating" section to do your planning.

3. **Advertise carefully when it is through non-personal means.**
   Make your advertising dollars count. Your advertising budget can be as much as 20% of gross for a new practitioner for the first 18 months. Then it averages about 10% per month for established practitioners.

Overadvertising can be as dangerous as underadvertising, advertising in an obscure part of a publication, advertising in an unrelated publication for your target market, or having poor advertising.

Remember that presentation is far more cost-effective and more powerful than advertising. So put your energies there. Advertising, however, is necessary for building name recognition. Excellent advertising well positioned in the right publications with photo and articles can be impactive in generating new patients. Get professional advice before you present your advertising. To keep your advertising spending in perspective, remember that practices build primarily through personal contact, educating patients and others about you. Generally, 75% of a practitioner's new patients are by referral.

4. **Don't overanticipate by overbuying or overstocking.**
This applies to equipment, health care products for sale, forms, office supplies. Buy what is appropriate now. Focus on quality care with simplicity. You are not out to impress with overextended affluence. It will only create anxiety and contraction which will keep your patients away.

5. **Carefully make income generating and image building expenses which invite or raise cash flow.**
New or like new carpet, paint, a few flowers and trimmed landscape attract! A worn carpet or unpainted walls and unkempt landscape show lack of care and detract. No need to overimpress, however. If it is a matter of attraction or detraction, it's basic. Taking care of it will serve you many times over.

An expense which neither adds nor attracts particularly can wait. Don't buy equipment which yields low income at the beginning of a practice. It's a luxury you can't afford.

6. **Utilize best what you have, and purchase what you don't have and need.**
If your equipment and furniture can be upgraded by paint or polishing, make it as up to date as possible. Check with other acupuncturists in the area for equipment purchasing, rather than buying new, if you need to save on finances.

Your diagnostic and treating equipment should be as state of the art as possible. Invest well.

Use the Focus forms. Photocopy clean copies of forms. It reflects on your image. Put some on colored paper. It brightens up the atmosphere and that has value. Or, for finest quality, use printed forms.

7. **Stretch your dollar and your payments as needed.**
Put minimum deposits where needed, pay on time until cash flow increases. Increase the size of payment in percentage to your income increase and pay where you receive discounts. Take loans where it's more advantageous than to purchase items outright, which in turn will expand your business and earn funds faster than the interest rate on your loans. Spend proportionately.

8. **Allow for seasonal variations in expenses.**
Monthly, quarterly and annual tax payments are irregular. Promotional expenses, insurance prepayments, professional fees, inventory replacements, loan repayments --these may all come due in different amounts in different months. They may come due in appalling large bunches. Seasonal income may vary considerably unless you do specific marketing to offset a normal seasonal services slump. Allow for the disproportion in income and expenses. Don't get caught short now because the month prior you thought you had extra funds to buy that new piece of equipment you have been longing to purchase.

9. **Professional fees and payroll must yield a good return for your investment.**
Do you need to outlay additional expense in excellent help to get the quality and build the practice you need? Is the number of hours you pay for assistance fit your practice needs right now? Should greater expense and hours or less expense and hours be outlaid?

10. **Pay payroll and quarterly taxes in a timely way so you avoid additional penalty charges.**

11. **Set aside contingency funds.**
Depending on your situation, contingency funds should be banks for from six months to 18 months. Set aside funds for emergency situations, seasonal variation in income, as well as for income and payroll taxes.

Start Up, Maintenance, Renovation, and Expansion Cost Estimating

After testing your awareness of the financial impact of your decisions, get very realistic with your figures. Considerable financial estimating will need to be done regrading financing, maintaining, or expanding your practice. You will need to do some research to start your practice and run your practice successfully.

You can fill in some of the estimates and discern some of the financial impact of your decisions by contacting:

❑ Health care needs and fees of the area by contacting other like services and the Department of Health in the area of consideration.

❑ Commercial brokers regarding rent, lease and purchase costs, leasehold improvement, and taxes for office space in the area.

❑ Utility costs from landlords as you investigate office space.

❑ Cost of living index of the area, demographics, and the expansion of the area by contacting the Chamber of Commerce.

❑ Professional equipment supplies from acupuncture equipment suppliers and by contacting other acupuncturists for good used equipment they may be selling.

❑ Office forms companies regarding the cost of bookkeeping and printing forms.

❑ Office supply stores concerning the cost of bulk rate office supplies or supplies bought on a revolving charge account.

❑ Insurance through your acupuncture associations or through an insurance broker or brokers.

❑ Signs should be checked with both a sign company after checking with the local architect review board for permissibility.

❑ Advertising costs. Compare the benefits of different ways, types, and costs of advertising by meeting with an advertising agency. Speak with your telephone book advertising companies, as well as the local newspaper advertising department.

❑ Consulting fees. Check with the bar association for lawyers. Talk with accountants, bookkeepers, and other health professionals. Use the "Practice Management Control Form" in the *Big Forms Packet*

An accountant/financial planner and practice management consultant can in the long run save you time and provide cost-saving connections with qualified professionals. (He/she) can analyze the best systems from which you can choose, and show you ways to outreach effectively. This type of consultant can save you from costly management errors, and help you plan or implement your budget, as well as provide guidance for you in expanding your services and profit.

What to Estimate

- 1. Cost, projections, and inventory.
  Overestimate expenses, underestimate income. Plan a contingency factor for the unknown. Fill in:

  Income and Expansion Balance Sheets
  1. Projection 6-12 month business income from services
  2. Income and expenses ratio sheets
  3. Projected and actual inventory of health product to sell
  4. Your break even and profit point

  Worksheets for Office Set-Up and Expansion Planning:
  5. The basics for establishing an acupuncture office
  6. Reception room front office, consultation room furniture and equipment start-up and expansion estimates and planning
  7. Professional equipment start-up and expansion planning and estimates

  Overall Totals
  8. Projected initial opening expenses
  9. Projected monthly practice expenses
  10. Personal expense sheet
     Start-up phase – start to the first 18 months. Plan to have other income source from outside. Don't expect income to live on fromyourpractice during this time.
  11. Management Control Form #5
     Balance sheet of assets and liabilities

- 2. Plan financial management control from the start.

  - ■ Projection of acute care/chronic type of patient balance, turnover (see Income Picture, page 118)

  - ■ Management Control Form #1
    Appointment and collection management control

  - ■ Management Control Form #2
    Shows review of day, week, and month of patient number, fees, accounts receivable status

■ Management Control Form #3
Projection of cash flow, type of account receivables, number of new patients per months, % from type of services, projected gross, taxes, and NET income *after* taxes.

■ Management Control Form #4
Yearly comparison of income and breakdown from type of services rendered, patient volume, #new patients, % collections, income comparison from month to month sheet.

3. Total Costs of Office Space
    ■ Initial: _____
    ■ Preparing for growth phase:_____
    ■ Preparing for expansion phase:_____
    ■ What costs can be reduced: _____
    _____
    _____
    _____
    _____
    _____

4. Fees and financial policies and points in time when you will review them.
    ■ Initial survey of fees:_____
    ■ Fee and financial policy review yearly basis (date):_____
    ■ Before planned growth phase:_____
    ■ Expansion phase: _____
    ■ Moving from primarily quantity practice to fewer patients more depth care: _ _____

5. Preparation of an initial marketing and expansion plan with cost projections before or during the following stages of practice:
    ■ Initial costs to 18 months: _____
    ■ Stabilization to growth phase: _____
    ■ Growth phase: _____
    ■ Expansion phase: _____
    ■ Leveling off phase: _____

•   In the Big Forms Packet

Establishing An Acupuncture Office (Basics)

(See extensive list in the Appendix)	Initial Expense	Monthly Expense

Furniture & Large Equipment
- Practitioner's Desk
- Chairs - Reception Room, Other
- Sectional couch
- Table
- Bookcase
- File cabinets
- Treatment Room equipment & supplies*

Furnishings
- Carpet
- Window coverings
- Pictures
- Plants (3)
- Lamps
- Literature/Magazine Racks
- Other _____

Office Supplies
- Folders
- Paper
- Pens
- Checks
- Bookkeeping System & Supplies
- Stamps
- Other _____

Professional Supplies
- Acupuncture Equipment*
- Acupuncture Supplies*
- Business Cards
- Appointment Book and Pages
- Stationary
- Planning Calendar
- Forms (Big Forms & Insurance Packet)
- Other _____

Establishing an Acupuncture Office (continued)

	Initial Expense	Monthly Expense
Office Equipment		
Typewriter	_____	_____
Phone (set-up and system)	_____	_____
Copier (	_____	_____
Water dispenser -- hot/ cold, teas, cups	_____	_____
Refrigerator	_____	_____
Answering machine	_____	_____
Other _____	_____	_____
Advertising		
Brochure	_____	_____
Yellow Pages Ad	_____	_____
Newspaper and other Publications	_____	_____
Other _____	_____	_____
Insurance		
Malpractice	_____	_____
Premises Liability	_____	_____
Medical	_____	_____
Disability	_____	_____
Other _____	_____	_____
Services		
Accounting/Bookkeeping	_____	_____
Secretarial	_____	_____
Phone Answering	_____	_____
Janitorial	_____	_____
Legal	_____	_____
Collections	_____	_____
Banking, Lease-hold, loan services	_____	_____
Utilities	_____	_____
Other _____	_____	_____
Facility		
Rent	_____	_____
Mortgage	_____	_____
Other _____	_____	_____

Inventory Supplies for Patient Sales

DESCRIPTION	INITIAL COST	MONTHLY COST	WHEN YOU WILL GET IT
Herbs			
☐ _____	_____	_____	_____
☐ _____	_____	_____	_____
☐ _____	_____	_____	_____
☐ _____	_____	_____	_____
☐ _____	_____	_____	_____
☐ _____	_____	_____	_____
☐ _____	_____	_____	_____
Supplements or Vitamins			
☐ _____	_____	_____	_____
☐ _____	_____	_____	_____
Supports			
☐ Neck supports, small	_____	_____	_____
☐ Cervical Pillows	_____	_____	_____
☐ Car or back supports	_____	_____	_____
☐ Wrist, elbow, knee, thigh, loin supports and belts - with or without magnet	_____	_____	_____
☐ Pregnancy support belts	_____	_____	_____
☐ Exercisers	_____	_____	_____
☐ Creams, salves, etc.	_____	_____	_____
☐ Cold packs (colpac)	_____	_____	_____
☐ Disposable self heating hot packs	_____	_____	_____
Other _____	_____	_____	_____
☐ Magnetic jewelry - necklaces, bracelets, anklets, earrings	_____	_____	_____
☐ Magnet cushions	_____	_____	_____
☐ Magnet shoes and insoles	_____	_____	_____
Other _____	_____	_____	_____

Projected monthly income from sales: _____

Total Practice Equipment and Supplies List

DESCRIPTION	INITIAL COST	MONTHLY COST	WHEN YOU WILL GET IT
Entrance & Reception Room			
Entrance			
☐ Exterior Professional Sign			
☐ Welcome Mat *"Take a step to health"*			
☐ Sign -- Name, Hours on your Door			
Basics			
☐ Chairs (6)			
☐ End Table (s) and or circle table			
☐ Lamps (2)			
☐ Educational Literature Racks			
☐ Shades or Draperies			
☐ Carpet (practical color, pleasing, durable, in good shape)			
☐ Heater (colder climate)			
☐ Fans / air-conditioning (hotter climate)			
☐ Water Dispenser /water, cups			
☐ Extra -- hot water urn, herb tea, etc			
Reputation and Image Builders			
☐ Take home Literature on Acupuncture Benefits,* Preventative care, Your maintenance program, We Love Referrals, * Your Specialty *(Big Forms Packet)			
☐ Placque that conveys your purpose			
☐ Pictures that convey your feeling tone and message			
☐ White or Colored Bulletin Board with removable or add or plastic letters for your messages about classes, your purpose, people who have referred			
☐ Displayed Articles -- written or items, (oriented for particular Patient Type)			
☐ Testimonial and Before-After Photo Book			
☐ Magazine Rack with the below:			

DESCRIPTION	INITIAL COST	MONTHLY COST	WHEN YOU WILL GET IT

Reception Room (Continued)

- ☐ Magazines for Specialty market, other
- ☐ Kiddie Corner w/Quiet Toys, Games or Magazines
- ☐ Patient Questionnaire on Service* (Big Forms Packet)

Tone Setters

- ☐ Plants (3)
- ☐ Stereo System with taped music
- ☐ Aquarium
- ☐ Mini-Waterfall Set-Up
- ☐ Fireplace
- ☐ Art Objects, Crystals, Sculptures

Front Office

Front Desk Area Furniture & Assecories

- ☐ Wide area desk --preferrably built in, long, L shape, or adaptable to increase work area, plenty of drawers
- ☐ Comfortable chair(s)
- ☐ Shelving
  (*see Records equipment storage*)
- ☐ Signs at front reception desk area:
  "Payment Due at the time services are rendered unless by prior arrangement"
  "Insurance Payment Plans Welcome"
  "Mastercard / Visa accepted" — No charge | No charge
- ☐ Extra Typewriter Table
- ☐ Computer Printer Table

Major Office Equipment

- ☐ Telephone (multiline 2-3 if possible -- with a hold botton & call hold and call forwarding ,)
- ☐ Intercom System - optional
- ☐ Answer box (beeper or dial in for messages type type)

DESCRIPTION	INITAL COST	MONTHLY COST	WHEN YOU WILL GET IT
☐ Answering machine tapes tapes outgoing -- emergency/special/lunch/ weekend/evening	_____	_____	_____
☐ Phone Pager	_____	_____	_____
☐ Adding machine with tape (a quiet one)	_____	_____	_____
☐ Typewriter (Preferably correcto-type)	_____	_____	_____
☐ Photocopy machine (or access to one)	_____	_____	_____
☐ Computer, hard disc, keyboard,	_____	_____	_____
☐ Computer screen and somashield,	_____	_____	_____
☐ Computer printer etc.	_____	_____	_____
Computer software packages			
☐ Accounting	_____	_____	_____
☐ Pagemaker -- for: newsletters, letters, advertising, marketing	_____	_____	_____
☐ Data Base - Mail order, etc.	_____	_____	_____
☐ Insurance Program	_____	_____	_____
☐ also for Diagnostic purposes	_____	_____	_____
☐ Other Computer equipment, fonts, etc.	_____	_____	_____
_____	_____	_____	_____
☐ Warranty and maintenance contracts	_____	_____	_____
☐ Recorder / Dictaphone (doing reports)	_____	_____	_____
☐ Big Clock (to keep on schedule)	_____	_____	_____

Records Equipment Storage

File Cabinets
-- For patient records
-- For Practitioner's office
-- For Front office forms & supplies
-- For oversized films

DESCRIPTION	INITAL COST	MONTHLY COST	WHEN YOU WILL GET IT
☐ 3-4 tier big file cabinet to go with file type you have pull-down front closes	_____	_____	_____
☐ 4 drawer, lettersize/ legal size	_____	_____	_____
☐ Short 2 drawer as above	_____	_____	_____
☐ File box (treatment card size) -- metal, compresses for fire protection	_____	_____	_____
☐ File box (ledger card size) -- metal, compresses	_____	_____	_____

DESCRIPTION	INITIAL COST	MONTHLY COST	WHEN YOU WILL GET IT

Printed Supplies ════════

☐ Appointment Book and Pages * (Big Forms Packet) _____ _____ _____

☐ Masters -- Big Forms Packet _____ _____ _____

☐ Masters -- Insurance Forms Packet _____ _____ _____

Printing Costs ════════

☐ Bulk Business Cards or Business Appointment card combination _____ _____ _____

☐ Forms (from existing masters) printed or photocopied _____ _____ _____

☐ Stationary with business name on it, plain paper for 2nd page _____ _____ _____

☐ Envelopes with business name on them _____ _____ _____

General Office Supplies *(One Time or Yearly)* ════════

☐ Business Card Holders

☐ To Do List and Weekly Plan List *(Volume II) _____ _____ _____

☐ Practitioner's Calendar _____ _____ _____

☐ Timer (quiet with pleasant buzz) for acuscope or tens machine _____ _____ _____

☐ Calendar (large and colorful) with scheduled office procedures such as for billing accounts payable/ monthly summary/staff meeting dates _____ _____ _____

☐ Log Book for New Patients _____ _____ _____

☐ Dictionary - English, Oriental, Spanish, Medical _____ _____ _____

☐ Acupuncture Referral Directory _____ _____ _____

Accounting & Billing System & Supplies ════════

☐ Receivable Control board/day sheets/deposit slips _____ _____ _____

☐ Record of procedures and charges (computerized or not)*(Big Forms Packet) _____ _____ _____

DESCRIPTION	INITIAL COST	MONTHLY COST	WHEN YOU WILL GET IT
☐ Acupuncturist's Fee-Communication Slip* (See Vol. II, Big Forms Packet)			
☐ Ledgers (Box listed above)			
☐ Ledger dividers at least 1-4 sets			
☐ Color coded dots for ledger financial plan coding			
☐ Billing envelopes			
☐ Mastercard/Visa machine from bank with minimal charge			
☐ Mastercard/Visa charge card slips (free)			

Accounts Payable System (computerized or not)

DESCRIPTION	INITIAL COST	MONTHLY COST	WHEN YOU WILL GET IT
☐ 1-write check writing system with distribution columns for overall operating expenses in office; includes checkbook with name, profession, professional address, phone number and social security or federal ID numbers.			
☐ Business Account Checks (if alone)			
☐ Expando files for accounts payable and paid			
☐ Cash box			

General Office Supplies Bulk

DESCRIPTION	INITIAL COST	MONTHLY COST	WHEN YOU WILL GET IT
☐ File folders (best with color coding)			
☐ Xerox paper (if you have a machine)			
☐ Other small and large paper			

Small Miscellaneous Office Supplies

DESCRIPTION	INITIAL COST	MONTHLY COST	WHEN YOU WILL GET IT
☐ Kwik stamp: name only _____, Licensed Acupuncturist			
☐ Kwik stamp: deposit to bank account, name, and number			
☐ Kwik stamp: Name, address, phone, tax identification number, Practice license number			
☐ Kwik stamp: "Benefits Assigned" stamp			

DESCRIPTION	INITIAL COST	MONTHLY COST	WHEN YOU WILL GET IT
☐ Stamp roll			
☐ Pencils			
☐ Pens			
☐ Pencil sharpener			
☐ Erasers			
☐ Colored Pencils			
☐ White out, pink, yellow, blue - to match paper			
☐ Correcto type			
☐ Stapler, staples remover, staples			
☐ Paper clips			
☐ Yellow, pink, or blue stick on squares for notes			
☐ Pads - for phone messages			
☐ Telephone log for long distance and insurance calls			
☐ Scissors			
☐ Letter opener			
☐ Hole punch			
☐ Scotch tape, masking, mailing tape			
☐ Date stamp and pad			
☐ Clip board			
☐ Letter moistener, ruler, ink pads			
☐ Rubber bands			
☐ Large and small thumb tacks			
☐ Rolodex and rolodex cards			

Larger Miscellaneous Equipment & Supplies

DESCRIPTION	INITIAL COST	MONTHLY COST	WHEN YOU WILL GET IT
☐ Refrigerator			
☐ File trays 2-3 tier			
☐ 5 tier on-the-wall file holder for patient histories, liens, boards, medical insurance information			
☐ Paper cutter (optional)			
☐ Bathroom supplies			
☐ Cleaning equipment vacuum cleaner, broom, quiet carpet sweeper dusting supplies, etc.			

Consultation Room

DESCRIPTION	INITAL COST	MONTHLY COST	WHEN YOU WILL GET IT
Furniture and Furnishings			
☐ Practitioner's Desk			
☐ Practitioner's Chair	_____	_____	_____
☐ Practitioner's File cabinet	_____	_____	_____
☐ Practitioner's Book case	_____	_____	_____
☐ Chairs (2-3)	_____	_____	_____
☐ Lucite Floor Mat	_____	_____	_____
Image Builders			
☐ Framed diplomas, items indicating excellence and recognition authority in the profession	_____	_____	_____
☐ Name plate and badge	_____	_____	_____
☐ Demonstration material	_____	_____	_____
☐ Plastic models, ear, hand, body, animal	_____	_____	_____
☐ Magnetic jewelry & shoes	_____	_____	_____
☐ Other _____	_____	_____	_____
☐ Educational pamphlets	_____	_____	_____
☐ Educational literature racks	_____	_____	_____
☐ Acupuncture wall chart	_____	_____	_____
☐ Viewer box (if you read films)	_____	_____	_____
☐ Displayed professional books	_____	_____	_____
☐ File stackers on desk (image: uncluttered and organized practitioner)	_____	_____	_____

Professional Equipment

DESCRIPTION	INITIAL COST	MONTHLY COST	WHEN YOU WILL GET IT

Treatment Room

Larger Treatment Room Items

	DESCRIPTION	INITIAL COST	MONTHLY COST	WHEN YOU WILL GET IT
☐	Treatment Table(s) (Portable)			
☐	Table Adjustment Board(s)			
☐	Treatment Table Paper			
☐	Table Pillows			
☐	Support Cushions -- back, leg, neck, wedges			
☐	Office Step Stool			
☐	Sitting Stool			
☐	Practitioner's Writing Table			
☐	Chair			
☐	Treatment Cart			
☐	Sterilization Equipment			
☐	(Autoclave, electric, steam, tubing, other; cleaning concentrates; glass bed sterilizers)			
☐	Acupuncture Charts and books			
☐	Other _____			
☐	Patient Cloth Gowns or Paper gowns			

Treatment Room Small Equipment

	DESCRIPTION	INITIAL COST	MONTHLY COST	WHEN YOU WILL GET IT
☐	Needle case			
☐	Needle storage vials			
☐	Bio Hazard Disposable Units for needles			
☐	Needle sterilizing container			
☐	Oxidation protective aids			
☐	Needle polishing			
☐	Needle sharpener			
☐	Scratching tools			
☐	Cryostim ice probe			
☐	Instrument tray			
☐	Kideny shaped basin			
☐	Waste bowls			
☐	Glass jars			

DESCRIPTION	INITIAL COST	MONTHLY COST	WHEN YOU WILL GET IT
☐ Stainless steel jars			
☐ Mortar and pestle			
☐ Moxa cup			
☐ Alcohol dispenser			
☐ Tweezers,			
☐ Forceps,			
☐ Skin tape			
☐ Scizzors			
☐ Thermometer and stand			
☐ Paper roll dispenser			
☐ Rubber stamps, labeling			
☐ Medical bag			
Disposable and Replaceables			
☐ Paper rolls			
☐ Cotton balls and swabs			
☐ Betadine swab aids			
☐ Acohol			
☐ Anticeptic pads			
☐ Self sealing sterilization pouches & tape			
☐ Incense sticks			
☐ Germicides			
☐ Tongue blades			
Examination and Diagnostic Equipment			
☐ Dermal & neurological hammers			
☐ Tuning, fork , pinwheel, accessories			
☐ Magnifers, tongue, ear, other			
☐ Penlight			
☐ Stethoscope			
☐ Sphygmomanometer			
☐ Kirlian equipment			
☐ Vega test with accompanying sample boxes			
☐ Entero machine			
☐ EAV instrument: dermatron or RMS 10			
☐ Acu-Data Electronic Oriental Acu-Therapy			
☐ Point detector			

DESCRIPTION	INITIAL COST	MONTHLY COST	WHEN YOU WILL GET IT

Needles

☐ (Bleeding, children's, cosmetic, disposable, Seirin, gold, Hinai-Shin Skin, Hwa To, Ido-No-Nippon-Sha, plum blossom, press tack, Enpi-Shin, prismatic, seven star, silver, silver handle, spring, super, Tai Chi, Chinese, veterinary, other)

☐ _____

☐ _____

☐ _____

Electro-Acupuncture Devices

☐ Japanese Ryodo-raku (with Meter Scales)

☐ Pointer F-3 Electro-Acupuncture, MEA, and TENS

☐ AWQ-100 Multi-Purpose Electronic Acupunctoscope

☐ Model IC-1103

☐ Acu-Polar 3B

☐ Haiky GK-3,

☐ El-Acupuncture,

☐ FY Apparatus

☐ Hand Held Point Locators

☐ Piezo Quartz Crystal Stim

☐ Acu-Lab-Electro-Acupuncture

☐ Ion Beam

☐ Model HP TENS

☐ HM-12 Massage Stimulator

☐ TX-2 and TX-3 TENS, batteries and Rechargers

☐ Dr Pulse

☐ Mini-M TENS, & Scalp Eletrode

☐ Connecting Wires for Needles and Accessories

☐ Magnetic and Electrode Probes

☐ Electrode Probes and TENS Accessories

☐ TENS Electrodes and Accessories

☐ Laser Apparatus,   Device

☐ WQ-10-B and C devices

☐ Executive Scan Cards

☐ Other _____

DESCRIPTION	INITIAL COST	MONTHLY COST	WHEN YOU WILL GET IT
Moxa and Moxibustion Equipment			
☐ Indirect Ibuki Moxa			
☐ Indirect Stick-On Moxa			
☐ Moxa accessories			
☐ Akabane devices			
☐ Loose and packaged Moxa & access.			
☐ Traditional and smokeless Moxa rolls			
☐ Electric Moxa and Moxa accessories			
Magnetic & Cutaneous Devices			
☐ Skin press pellets, Acupatches, and Acu-aids			
☐ Magnets			
☐ TDK BioMagnetic necklace and bracelets			
☐ Magnetic belts and magnetic supports			
☐ Wrist, elbow, knee, ankle supporters with magnets			
☐ Pregnancy support belts & manaka devices			
☐ Glass & plastic cupping sets & special devices			
☐ Cutaneous probes			
☐ Children's Shoni-Shin			
☐ Cutaneous rolling devices			
☐ Shoni-Shin			
Other Therapy Equipment			
☐ Ultrasound machine			
☐ Hydrocollator			
☐ Packs and covers			
☐ Hot packs (disposable, self-heating)			
☐ Cold packs (colpac) disposable			
☐ Refrigerator			

Projected Total Initial Opening Expenses

LEASEHOLD IMPROVEMENTS. . . . . $_____

RENT OR LEASE DEPOSIT . . . . $_____

EQUIPMENT LEASE DEPOSIT . . . . $_____

UTILITIES DEPOSITS. . . . . $_____

TELEPHONE DEPOSITS. . . . . $_____

PROFESSIONAL SUPPLIES . . . . $_____

BOOKKEEPING SYSTEM. . . . . $_____

INITIAL PRINTING. . . . . $_____

OFFICE SUPPLIES . . . . $_____

INSURANCE DEPOSITS. . . . . $_____

ADVERTISING & PROMOTIONS. . . . .$_____

PROFESSIONAL SIGN (if not in equipment lease) . . . .$_____

PERSONAL EXPENSES UNTIL PROJECTED OPENING DATE. . . . .$_____

CONSULTING FEES . . . .$_____

FRONT OFFICE STAFF (if warranted) . . . . $_____

_____ . . . . $_____

_____ . . . . $_____

TOTAL INITIAL OPENING EXPENSES. . . . . $_____

MY PROJECTED OPENING DATE IS

_____

Projected Monthly Practice Expenses

OFFICE RENT OR LEASE . . . . $_____

UTILITIES. . . . . $_____

EQUIPMENT LEASE. . . . . $_____

OPERATING LOAN & INTEREST. . . . . $_____

SALARIES - EMPLOYEES . . . . $_____

LEGAL FEES AND MANAGEMENT CONSULTING FEES. . . . . . $_____

ACCOUNTING OR BOOKKEEPING. . . . . $_____

OFFICE SUPPLIES. . . . . $_____

PROFESSIONAL SUPPLIES. . . . . $_____

INSURANCE (DISABILITY & OFFICE OVERHEAD) . . . .$_____

INSURANCE (MALPRACTICE). . . . . $_____

INSURANCE (LIFE, LIABILITY & PROPERTY DAMAGE). . . . . . $_____

TAXES-PAYROLL & OTHER. . . . . $_____

PROMOTION & ADVERTISING. . . . . $_____

CONVENTIONS & MEETINGS . . . . $_____

TELEPHONE & YELLOW PAGES . . . . $_____

DUES & SUBSCRIPTIONS . . . . $_____

MISCELLANEOUS. . . . . $_____

TOTAL PROJECTED EXPENSES . . . . $_____

Projected Monthly Personal Expenses

RENT.. $_____

UTILITIES.. $_____

GROCERIES....................................... $_____

INSURANCE....................................... $_____

AUTOMOBILE EXPENSES...................... $_____

MEDICAL EXPENSES............................ $_____

CLOTHING... $_____

DRY CLEANING.................................. $_____

TAXES... $_____

CREDIT LINES................................... $_____

DONATIONS....................................... $_____

CHILD CARE...................................... $_____

ENTERTAINMENT................................ $_____

MISCELLANEOUS................................ $_____

OTHER... $_____

TOTAL PROJECTED EXPENSES.............. $_____

Management Control Form #5

Profit And Loss Statement

Balance Sheet For

_____
(name of your firm)

As of _____
(date)

Assets

Current assets:
Cash:
Cash in bank .... $_____
Petty cash .... $_____
Accounts receivable .... $_____
Less allowance for doubtful accounts .... $_____
Merchandise inventories .... $_____
Total current assets .... $_____
Fixed assets:
Land .... $_____
Buildings .... $_____
Delivery equipment .... $_____
Furniture and fixtures .... $_____
Less allowance for depreciation .... $_____
Leasehold improvements, less amortization .... $_____
Total fixed assets .... $_____
Total assets .... $_____

Liabilities and Capital

Current liabilities:
Accounts payable .... $_____
Notes payable, due within 1 year .... $_____
Payroll taxes and withheld taxes .... $_____
Sales taxes .... $_____
Total current liabilities .... $_____
Long-term liabilities:
Notes payable, due after 1 year .... $_____
Total liabilities .... $_____
Capital:
Proprietor's capital, beginning of period .... $_____
Net profit for the period .... $_____
Less proprietor's drawings .... $_____
Increase in capital .... $_____
Capital, end of period .... $_____
Total liabilities and capital .... $_____

Total Assets .... $_____
Total Liabilities .... Less$_____
Net Worth .... $_____

PM112 (c) 1986 C. Flint

PROJECTION OF INCOME FROM SERVICES RENDERED

Month	Week	No. Of New Pts.	No. Of Est. Pts.	Examinations	Treatment	Other				Total
1	1									
	2									
	3									
	4									
	Total									
2	1									
	2									
	3									
	4									
	Total									
3	1									
	2									
	3									
	4									
	Total									
4	Total									
5	Total									
6	Total									
7	Total									
8	Total									
9	Total									
10	Total									
11	Total									
12	Total									

Total First Year Projected Income: $ _____

EXPENSES WORKSHEET

BALANCE FORWARD:
EXPECTED INCOME:
10 % MONEY MAGNET:

ACCT. NO.	DESCRIPTION	1	2	3	4	5	6	7	8	9	10	11	12
426	INSURANCE - GROUP												
428	INSURANCE - WORKERS' COMPENSATION												
429	MEETINGS AND SEMINARS												
430	OUTSIDE SERVICES - CLERICAL												
431	OUTSIDE SERVICES - MEDICAL												
432	OUTSIDE SERVICES - DATA PROCESSING												
438	PROFESSIONAL FEES												
442	RENT - EQUIPMENT												
444	RENT - REAL ESTATE												
450	REPAIRS AND MAINTENANCE												
454	SALARIES AND WAGES												
462	SUPPLIES - OFFICE												
464	SUPPLIES - HERBS												
465	SUPPLIES - OTHER												
470	TAXES - PAYROLL												
472	TAXES - PROPERTY												
476	TAXES AND LICENSES												
480	TELEPHONE												
486	TRAVEL AND ENTERTAINMENT												
492	UNIFORMS												
494	UTILITIES												
496	VEHICLE OPERATIONS (PRACTITIONER'S)												
499	MISCELLANEOUS												
991	INTEREST:												
1000	PERSONAL												
	SUBTOTAL :												
	TOTAL INCOME:												
	TOTAL EXPENSES:												
	NET PROFIT:												NET PROFIT MOS. PER.

PM104B (c) 1987 C. Flint

EXPENSES WORKSHEET

BALANCE FORWARD:
EXPECTED INCOME:
10 % MONEY MAGNET:

ACCT. NO.	DESCRIPTION	1	2	3	4	5	6	7	8	9	10	11	12
101	MONEY-IN-BANK - CHECKING												
103	MONEY-IN-BANK - SAVINGS												
104	PETTY CASH												
143	LEASEHOLD IMPROVEMENTS												
144	ACCUMULATED DEPRECIATION - L.I.												
145	EQUIPMENT												
146	ACCUMULATED DEPRECIATION - EQUIPMENT												
147	VEHICLES												
148	ACCUMULATED DEPRECIATION - VEHICLES												
242	NOTES PAYABLE												
243	CONTRACT PAYABLE												
290	CAPITAL												
299	DRAW												
300	INCOME - PROFESSIONAL FEES												
302	INCOME - OTHER												
402	ADVERTISING AND PROMOTION												
405	ANSWERING SERVICE												
406	AUTO EXPENSE (EMPLOYEES)												
407	BANK CHARGES												
408	BONUSES												
416	DEPRECIATION EXPENSE												
417	DONATIONS												
418	DUES AND SUBSCRIPTIONS												
419	EMPLOYEE BENEFITS												
424	INSURANCE - CASUALTY												
	SUBTOTAL:												
	TOTAL INCOME:												
	TOTAL EXPENSES:												
	NET PROFIT:												NET PROFIT MOS. PER.

PM104A (c) 1987 C. Flint

6 MONTH INCOME PROJECTION

MONTH:

WEEK:	Projected	Actual	Projected	Actual	Projected	Actual	Projected	Actual	Projected	Actual	Projected	Actual
Week #1 INCOME												
EXPENSES												
Week #2 INCOME												
EXPENSES												
Week #3 INCOME												
EXPENSES												
Week #4 INCOME												
EXPENSES												
Week #5 INCOME												
EXPENSES												
MONTHLY TOTALS: INCOME												
EXPENSES												
Amount Increased												

The Break Even and Profit Formula for Practices

You must be able to assess what your break-even point is and what it will take to profit if you are to stay in practice. The following is a formula to use for this purpose.

■ First, Look at the chart on "Where Much of An Office Visit Fee Goes." These are fixed expenses. Your variable expenses are things such as marketing supplies and advertising, long distance phone, remedies which are part of treatment, travel, entertainment, donations. Variable costs are not necessarily expendable costs. Marketing, for example is vital to practice expansion; so make sure you have open ended procedures set up and a specific action oriented expansion and marketing plan. You wouldn't want to find yourself with a fully set up office, procedures in place, but very little to fill it while the rent and overhead continues to run because of a poor or no marketing plan. Nor would you want expansive marketing to create a large influx of people with a poorly set up practice with scattered and unclear procedures. This would turn the patients off once they came to your office, and decrease both patient and financial returns.

■ Second, look at your "Expenses Worksheets." Separate your costs into two kinds: fixed and variable.

■ Third, use the estimated "Income and Expense Projection Worksheets" to estimate cash flow over the next 6-12 months.

■ Fourth, figure your total costs per month. Breakdown your total expenses for the year so they can be handled over 12 months.

■ Fifth, know the usual, reasonable and customary rate for your services in your area, and figure the bottom line you must charge to break even, expand, and/or meet your profit goal. What is your bottom line charge for services? Your top end charge for services?

1. **How many patient visits must you have per month to break even?** (N) Number of pt. visits per month = (F) Monthly Fixed cost divided by [($)Fee for service - (V) Variable costs broken down per pt. visit). Now add (I) 1/2 patient visit per every visit you intend to do part insurance assignment.

   You must calculate both your (PFE) practice fixed expenses and your (PE) personal expenses into your fixed costs if you will make it financially. You also must allow for (I) moneys to be outstanding because of insurance assignment or billing arrangements.

2. **How much must you make to meet your personal expenses and profit?**

   This is your break even profit formula. Multiply (N) the number of non-insurance patient visits plus (I) 1/2 number of insurance patient visits. Multiply times [($) the usual standard price for services minus (V) the total variable cost (broken down per visit)]. Then subtract (PFE +PE) total fixed costs.

$$Profit = [(N - I) \times (\$ - V)] - [PFE + PE]$$

What parts of your financial, operational, and marketing plan can be adjusted to work better for you? Is additional money needed? Project if you will need a larger loan or any changes in your practice to reduce expenses. Use a profit and loss statement each month or quarterly statements. Invest in sold advice from a good practice management consultant, accountant, lawyer, and lender who has not been involved in your working out the daily details may be able to see the weaknesses that failed to appear as you poured over details. They may be able to bring out the strong points of your plan that you should emphasize.

What Is Your Plan for Getting Funded?

1. What are your reasons for needing funding?

_____

_____

_____

_____

2. What do you want to do? For each goal figure the amount needed
   and the per cent needed of your total budget.

SHORT RANGE GOALS	%	$ AMT
Monthly fixed expenses		
Other:		

BUDGET LONG RANGE GOALS	%	$ AMT

3. How much money do you want (TOTAL)? _____
   (Underestimate income and overestimate expenses). Figure no less than 6 months expenses.

4. How long will it take you to accomplish what you want?
   (Allow for the unexpected. Ask yourself: How long do you usually imagine things take to accomplish? How long do they realistically tend to take? Allow for the realistic approach.)

   _____
   _____
   _____
   _____

5. How much debt do you want to handle each month and for how long?

   _____
   _____

6. How will you put money aside for repayment? Special savings account? Time payments? Other _____

7. How long will it take you to repay your debts on the course you have directed for yourself? How will you put aside for it?

   _____
   _____
   _____
   _____
   _____

8. What form of borrowing is the most efficient, effective means for what you want? _____

   _____

❏ **Be aware of problems in borrowing:**

1. Not being able to speak to the person who does the lending.
2. Having inadequate records or proof of financial stability.
3. Establishing credit. No credit record.
4. Frequent changing of jobs or location.
5. Possible delays in getting approval for funds, actually receiving the funds, which would hold up leasing office space, buying equipment, etc.
6. _____

❏ **And opportunities in borrowing!**

Borrowing creates leverage, which can be valuable for your future needs. Remember: Debt is not bad. Just use it wisely and plan well! Have your plan reviewed. If you need them, the Small Business Association has free service advisors. What a loan is: Money you get to use, and promise to pay back at a later date with principal and usually interest. It's advisable to prepare for some form of loan.

These are questions to ask your banker: What determines the rate of interest? What is the prime rate? What are compensating balances? How can leveraging help you? What are the types of bank loans you could use?

1. Commercial: (secured or unsecured)
2. Installment: (monthly payment plus interest)
3. Passbook: (Low risk)
4. Accounts receivable:
5. Factoring?
6. Real estate (construction and takeout): ,
7. Small Business Administration Guaranteed:

How to Present Your Practice Plan
When You Apply for A Loan

The following is a list of what to present when applying for a loan. This should be in writing. This shows you are professional and that you know how to plan. You want to reinforce your strengths, your ability to plan, carry out planning, and convince the lender that you are a good risk.

1. **Your purpose** in practicing acupuncture.

2. The purpose for the **use of the funds**—itemized list and cost projections.

3. **Source of repayment**--what services you offer; projections for expansion of services — fee structure, income and expense projections.

4. **Character and stability.** Show experience in running a business; the last 2-3 years of tax returns; a willingness to be in one place; long term employment or residency; a willingness to pay; past experience of repaying loans; background of service/honorability.

5. Primary and secondary **assets.** Submit a financial current statement.

6. **Collateral** . Show your ability to repay —i.e. items that can be borrowed against and liquidated, if there is a need.

7. **Ability to make a profit.** Present profit and loss statements.

8. The condition of the **market place** - Convey the national and local average of earnings in this profession if it is to your benefit. The most recent survey can be obtained from the survey done by Redwing and CAA or national associations.

9. **Access** to facilities which you are considering leasing or buying; access to records if you are considering buying a practice, or access to an appraiser's records; available information on the rate of business growth in this general area or locale.

In presenting your practice plan, it is important to ask yourself, what does a lender look at in a request for a credit accommodation?

The 5 C's of credit the bank looks for:
1. Character
2. Capacity
3. Capital
4. Collateral
5. Condition of the market place

How to Prepare for a Loan Interview.

Include:
❑ 1. One page of information on you and your experience in busi ness.
❑ 2. Two year end statements; the last two years of tax returns.
❑ 3. Cash flow projections for the next 6-12 months.
❑ 4. Suitable security.
❑ 5. Credit History.
❑ 6. Their loan application filled out.
❑ 7. Be aware of the problems in borrowing and ask about the opportunities.

Fill out a Credit Application

❑ l. Write to the bank, finance or leasing companies and get an application.

❑ 2. Include your practice plan as outlined .

OVERVIEW

A Realistic Financial Picture of Cash Flow, Management and Profit

Most healers by nature tend to be service-oriented, and a good number are optimists. Optimism must be balanced by practicality. Because practice stability is so vital, particularly in the beginning stages, overoptimism can mean certain death to the practice. To be successful in practice, a practitioner-owner/manager must be able to see the financial impact of his choices and decisions for the practice to stabilize, grow, and expand. The financial planning and management section provides a good basis from which to understand the financial implications of your choices. The "Pitfalls to Avoid for Successful Practice" and the section on "Monitoring your Practice" at the end of the book can help guide you as well.

However, when you have filled in your financial plan, still take it to a good accountant or financial planner in the beginning <u>before</u> you leap. Remember: feedback is a necessary ingredient of success. Good practice planning <u>and</u> professional advice can avoid problems later!

How can you best be prepared? In a new business, have sufficient cash to start and take you through the cash flow deficits of the first 6-18 months of operation. One of the biggest dangers is overestimating income and underestimating expenses. This occurs because practitioners are new at their practice, really don't know their business, haven't given it enough thought, or are simply overoptimistic. Cash overruns are not something which just happen. So aside from an awareness of the financial impacts of your decisions, one of your biggest safeguards is to build into your capital budget a substantial contingency reserve to cover you in the beginning of your practice. You can avoid the number one failure of practices, which is undercapitalized from the start. Take a longer time if necessary to open your practice on a solid financial basis, rather than to plunge in and continually do crisis management because of underplanning and undercapitalizing.

Because the record keeping system is your means for keeping your practice on track, you will want to set this up before your practice opens so you can track your practice from day one. If you do it later, you may be too busy to give the record keeping system the proper attention.

Responsibility for cash management starts with calculated estimates of cash inflows and cash outflow, as well as accurate recording. You have started on a solid foundation by doing the estimates in this section. Be aware that practices may show a profit, but still have cash flow problems. You will need to "mange cash flow." This is simply planning for the balance or correcting the difference between incoming cash and outgoing cash at the end of a particular time period.

Understand the way profit works. *Profit* is the way accountants describe the fee to be paid by a patient which is matched against the commitments made by you to pay expenses. But the actual way we transact business does not reflect this. Income is not the same as cash receipts. Expenses are not the same as actual cash expenditures. They occur at different times. In short, the profits are booked after the expenditures, but before the patient's payments are received. There is an outflow of cash before the corresponding inflow. In fact, the cash disbursements for labor, inventory, overhead, and other expenses necessary to produce or provide services may precede by two to three months or more the actual cash receipts in payment for those services and products, especially when liberal credit terms are extended. For a potentially decisive period of time, there are significant outflows of cash, but little inflow.

Also be aware that there are a number of ways which profits may not generate equal amounts of cash available for current operations.

1. Tax obligations must be set aside. Hence, precash profits do not yield equal amounts of cash.

2. Loans or advances must be repaid.

3. Expenses occurring in irregularly large clumps combined with low income months can upset cash flow.

4. Profits may be reinvested into the practice, which decrease cash.

One of the practitioner's biggest jobs in the role of financial manger is to make sure the cash flow is controlled and income and expenses are proportionate to pay the expenses and make a profit. This takes timing and balancing the inflows and outflows of funds. As we have discussed, anticipate cash will be available to meet those needs on a very timely basis. Plan for cycles of increase and decrease so increasing periods cover periods of decrease in income. If financial management is not your forte, hire a good accountant or financial advisor to assist you. You can specify your needs to an accountant, and he can help you with any of the following:

1. Help set up an appropriate accounting system and show you how to make the most of it.

2. Help organize and supervise in-house staff in the keeping of books to avoid unwitting chaos.

3. Provide timely, accurate, and useful financial statements so you can understand what's going on.

4. Make sure appropriate financial controls are in place so you don't squander cash and other assets.

5. Help detect theft before it cripples your practice.

6. Prepare accurate and timely tax returns that give you advantages of all legitimate savings and help in advance with both practice and personal tax planning.

7. Experienced in small business operating problems, a well-recommended accountant can give you valuable advice on running your practice.

Your assistant can help you by using the "Management Control Forms" in the *Big Forms Packet. A* good front office manager should be able to do an analysis for you on the statistics, particularly if he/she has read the factors discussed in the income and expense planning and management section.

The previous section has been devoted to a consideration of inflow and outflow planning, so your cash flow and income can be sufficient to maintain, grow and expand your practice, as well as profit! You know enough of a planning basis to move on and prepare for the next step, which is considering the best office space for you, how you choose it, set it up, and then operate in practice!

OFFICE SPACE

Preparing to Look for an Office

Recap your unique advantage which can most attract those who need what you do best: _____

_____

To what patient types, ages, conditions, socioeconomic groups am I most drawn or do I prefer to locate near? _____

_____

_____

Where can I best locate near those who are most responsive now to what I offer best ? _____

_____

Where can I best locate near those who can afford to compensate me for what I best offer? _____

_____

Where can my practice most easily or best stabilize? _____

_____

Where can my practice best grow? _____

_____

Where can I best locate with present and loan capabilities? _____

_____

Where can I best grow professionally and personally? _____

_____

Where can my personal and family needs be best balanced with professional goals? _____

Where can I best afford on all levels to locate? _____

_____

Where to Find Your Practice and Your Office Space

The best time to look for your practice space is when:

- You have explored and decided on an area in which to practice and have
  done a market research study on the area first.
- You are familiar with good location and office criteria described in this book.
- You have explored the type of arrangement(s) you must have: associate program; sharing space; buying a practice; starting from scratch in a home/office; renting or leasing; or buying a building.
- You have considered dhow you will fund your practice and your space.

Depending on the type of arrangement you want, various combinations of the below sources will be helpful to you in finding your best office space.

- 1. Newspaper classified advertising (for renting, leasing residential, commercial space. Put an ad in the locale of your choice (county, state or national publication) stating:

  Wanted: Office space in Medical building for acupuncture practice. xxx sq.ft. etc.
  Wanted: Commercial building for acupuncture practice
  Wanted: Duplex or Home/office combination near downtown _____(area).
  Contact: your name, address, and phone number.

- 2. Commercial brokers (for renting, leasing, or buying office space)

- 3. Look at existing classified ads in acupuncture professional publications (acupuncture association journals, newsletters) and create you own stating:

  Wanted: Associateship in acupuncture practice in _____(area).
  Wanted: Partnership in acupuncture practice in _____area.
  Wanted: Acupuncture Practice for sale in_____area.
  Contact: Name, address, phone, excellent references available.

■ 4. Look at existing classified ads in medical, chiropractic, specific health practitioner newsletters and add your classified:

Wanted: Acupuncturist wants to share office space with medical doctorin _____area. Excellent References. Contact: Name, Address, Phone.

■ 5. Contact acupuncture colleges to place an ad or find an ad on their bulletin boards for what you want.

■ 6. Contact the local society meeting, if there is any, to pick up leads on who wants to add staff, retire, sell their practice, or relocate.

■ 7. Contact leading acupuncturists in the area in which you want to practice.

■ 8. Get a copy of the Yellow Pages Telephone Directory for the entire area in which you want to practice. (You can usually photocopy the section you need from your local library directory.) Write or call the acupuncturists there. Ask them if they have or will be having an associateship position, partnership, practice for sale etc. If not, ask: "Do you know who does?" State that any information they share with you will be confidential. You should find out very quickly the status of availability.

■ 9. Contact president of the acupuncture society, locally or nationally, or at the state level.

■ 10. Practice management consulting businesses.

■ 11. Acupuncture suppliers—material and equipment.

■ 12. If you want to buy a practice, contact a practice broker, i.e. Professional Practice Sales in Southern and Northern California, Illinois, and New York. Before buying an existing practice, check under "Advantages and Disadvantages of Buying a Practice," in the manual and read *How to Buy and Sell a Practice* by Dr. Peter G. Fernandez.

Thoroughly check a number of possible locations. Your location is a big investment in your practice. If you have any questions or doubts regarding location and office space, one of your team--your practice consultant, your lender, your lawyer, your accountant--are able to assist you before you sign any agreements involving your practice space.

How to Decide on Your <u>Best</u> Office Space

Previously, we looked at being part of someone else's space and buying a practice. These have "already setup" spaces with policies included.*

We'll look at in this next section how you want to choose your space when you set up your practice from scratch. Your choices: Use a home/office combination; buy a building; or, rent/lease either sole or group shared office space. We'll compare them first and then look at the specifics on each one. Your choice is often based on economical and type of practice style considerations.

In all cases, you must know how to evaluate a good office space and how to go about arranging it. We've set it up in a form you can use to do this. Whatever you choose, don't sacrifice good location or quality. Get the best for your dollar.

---

* Agreements are in the *Big Forms Packet.*

Should I Have an Office away from Home?

The advantages of an out-of-home office are:[1]
1. It's considered more professional.
2. You can leave your work behind when you go home.
3. Calls come into the office, not your residence, unless you choose to have calls ring through to you, or you choose to use a pager.
4. Other professionals are nearby, particularly if you locate in a medical complex.
5. An office can have the image of credibility, of being established, more modern, up to date, state of the art , requiring competency and success.
6. Patients generally feel more secure coming to a professional health care office rather than a home.

Other advantages of shared office space:
7. Colleagues are available for consultation or second opinion at most times.
8. Expenses are shared.
9. You don't have to pay for a whole week of space. You can rent by the day or by hour.
10. Association with an established office brings you credibility.

The disadvantages of having your own professional office are:
1. Expensive rent and utilities, <u>unless</u> they are shared among others or you rent space by the day or hour.
2. Leases can be too long or too short and inflexible.
3. You generally must spend the day at the office.
4. You must furnish your own office which can be costly--unless of course, you are an associate in an associateship practice or in a partnership.

Additional disadvantages if you share your office or office rooms:
5. If you share rooms with other health practitioners, they may or may not be as neat or careful as you are.
6. Too many policies may not be compatible with your style.
7. You may not be able to use the facilities as freely as you would like.
8. Patients may prefer a quieter one practitioner office to a multiple practitioner office with a busy waiting room or front office staff who may not be trained to represent you as you would like.
9. You may not get your messages, personalized attention, or the proper attention to obtaining the new patient caller "shopping" for the right practitioner in a busier office, where front office staff is shared by many professional health care practitioners.

[1] Beck, Leif, C., *The Physician's Office*, Princeton, N..J. Excerpta Medica, 1977.

"If I Have a Home/Office Combination?"

Advantages

When you first start a practice, you may want to setup a home/office combination. If you do, be sure to check with local ordinances to make sure you can legally practice in a home. Some areas forbid medical practice in a home.

Whenever you start a practice, you have to consider total expenses, not only the expenses of running an acupuncture office. You must allow for taxes, inflation, and the total living expenses of owning a home or renting an apartment. If you have a home/office combination, you will reduce your total expenses by at least one-third. This might mean the difference between survival and failure.

If you are fortunate enough to locate a good home/office combination, (See advantages of locating.) Make sure your office is located in a way that your children won't distract your patients or the smell of food from the kitchen won't enter your office. A duplex is an excellent example of a good home/office combination. It also gives you room for expansion as your practice grows. It also might meet otherwise sticky legal requirements.

Availability of 24 hour service to your patients can be a real advantage in the beginning of a practice. This may not be attractive to you later, but in the beginning of your practice, this means business and serving people. By either installing an extension phone in your home or using a pager, you will be able to answer telephone calls that come in late evenings, on weekends, and over mealtime hours. Patients can come to you in your atmosphere, which can be an advantage or a disadvantage, depending on your situation. Other advantages: It's close and convenient. You can eliminate the cost, time, and aggravation of driving to and from another office space. It can be a warm and more comfortable environment for your patients, as long as it appears tastefully professional to your patient .

P 175 of "If I have a home/office combination? was primarily cited from Dr. Peter Fernandez's, How to Start a Practice From Scratch.

If a home/office combination is permissible for you, there are many tax deductions:

Rent	Homeowners" insurance
Repairs	Interest
Housecleaning	Utilities
Mortgages or loans	Business phone
Fence (protection)	Property protection-guard dog

The *"Business Use of Your Home"* is the proper form to use for tax purpose in recording these expenses. These expenses are totaled and a specific percentage can be deducted from your gross income on *Schedule C*. Keep accurate records and receipts. If you have an 8 room house and 4 are used for business purposes only, you can claim 50% of your expenses for business. Office furniture and equipment can be depreciated. See a tax advisor regarding deductions.

Disadvantages

The disadvantages are that patients can call and bother you during family hours and you and your family decrease your privacy. Your patients know more about you and your life-style. Also, a patient who acts out could potentially harm you or your home.

If I Decide to Rent or Lease Office Space. . .

■ 1. Decide your potential locations, how much space, and what kind of layout you want for:
A consulting room
Business and reception area
Toilet
Treatment room and dressing room combination(s)

Remember, practice patterns are not yet known and growth comes differently for each practitioner. In your final decision, make sure the reception area can accommodate twice the number of patients seen at peak hours.

■ 2. Decide how much you can afford. The percentage which total rental costs will bear to the practice's annual gross income is important. Average occupancy costs from 5%-8% of gross income. (Ibid. The ratio appropriate to you depends on what you can bear.) The ratio must be looked at with the practice's anticipated volume and income. Rental costs at the start may be as high as 20%. There are arguments for both renting and leasing smaller and larger space. Consider the following scenarios:

" I rented about 800 to 1,000 square feet, and planned on being so busy that I would need to move in three years. I didn't carry the rent on 1,500 square feet just so I would have it in three years. The extra overheads would have sunk me. Moving in three years was no big deal. In fact, it was a reason to public relate and advertise my successful growing practice."

Some practitioners lease a larger space than they need and rent those rooms out to other practitioners. This assures cash flow and phasing out rental space as your practice grows. This also prevents having to move. If you have prime location and a good lease, you wouldn't want to move.

■ 3. Find a couple of potential spaces.

■ 4. Review these spaces using the checklist following.

■ 5. Carefully examine the terms of the contract. Use the "Checklist" on the following pages to assist you.

We advise having an attorney check the lease for you. Leases are designed for the benefit of the landlord, not necessarily for the lessee. Find out what services besides square footage space are provided. Don't assume anything and make sure all services are in writing prior to signing the contract.

■ 6. Obtain and fill in a rental or lease "Condition and Inventory Checklist," which you can purchase through most stationary stores in their forms section. With your landlord, walk through the office you intend to lease, and note all conditions and inventory of the office site. At the time you sign your contract, keep one copy of the checklist with the contract for yourself and give one set to your landlord. This will insure a clear basis from which to assess the condition of the office when you vacate it.

Leases need to be negotiated with flexibility. Short-term leases with "options to renew" are best. A four year lease with two successive options to renew for three years each with rental increases of $.25 / per square foot is an example. This leaves the acupuncturist with a choice. A variety of escape clauses should be considered. Consider for example, is there payment of a penalty if the acupuncturist dies, is disabled or dissolves his partnership? How would you want to handle this? Consider the desirability of the right to sublet the office. Look at the owners or your own willingness to foot the bill for tenant improvements, such as soundproofing, partition construction or removal or outlets and lighting. Provisions for improvements or "redecoration (painting) and recarpeting" must be written into the lease. We emphasize, consult an attorney before signing a lease. It will save you problems now and in the long run.

"If I Want to Buy a Building...."

If you buy a building you have the advantage of fixing it up or creating your own environment and tax write offs. If you buy correctly, you can build in plans for expansion and resalability. In any case, if you decide to buy, contact an experienced and well-trusted real estate broker. Obtain a commercial properties broker who is not connected in any way with the seller of your potential building. He will know the selling prices of most commercial buildings, as well as rental and construction costs, the true value of the building, and if it is worth the purchase price. He will help look at the value of property (the area now and in the future), and he will help you negotiate the purchase. (Important: Check with a C.P.A. for tax advantages before settling on terms.) The broker will be familiar with zoning codes, and most important, with the people who write and administer them. The fact that a commercial business was located in a building doesn't necessarily mean that zoning regulations will allow an acupuncture office in that building. A good real estate broker can (probably more than anyone else) give you an accurate idea of total costs — from rewiring and remodeling to mortgage payments and taxes.

Allow for expansion. If you buy or build a clinic to fit your present requirements, it probably will change within the next five years. If you design a single-purpose building, it may be difficult to finance and even harder to sell. Design your building so that any business could use it. Movable partitions and non-weightbearing internal walls will change your building from single to a multiple purpose building and enhance resale and value.

"If I Want to Buy a Building" was primarily cited from Dr. Peter G. Fernandez's *How to Start and Practice from Scratch.*

Good Office Location

1, **Area Location** (see section on "The Value of Location").

2. **Practice in a "Zone" where people prefer to go.**
   If you want to practice in a large town, go toward the suburbs. Those in the suburbs don't want to drive through crowded traffic to get to their health practitioners. Also, if the health practitioners tend to group in an area and people are used to going there for health care, business activities, and grocery shopping, locate there. Shopping malls are often perfect. Go where the people go.

3. **Meets zoning requirements.**
   Are you in a zone where you can have a practice? Can you have adequate sign exposure and is parking readily available? Can you practice without arousing "looks" from neighbors or adjacent offices? Do you have excessive human or auto traffic coming to your office over and above the norm of the neighborhood? Can you insulate for smell, noise factors, as well as warmth? Is exposure of your practice in this location going to be any problem? If it is, you will go into contraction and limit your practice. Go where the surroundings will support you.

4. **Health care complex.**
   It is easier to refer next door and keep the lines of communication open if practitioners can easily access each other.

5. **Good traffic flow.**
   Look at a map. Locate the main arteries going in and out of the town. Where are the booming areas? Locate new areas, well-established areas, older and newer run-down areas.

   One successful practitioner states: "I have always tried to locate my office close to the business region of a city, about halfway home, and near a ring road. Usually there is an area where the freeways have been built, just outside the office blocks and high density daytime traffic. People living in suburbia can come in on uncongested roads and get on the ring road, and then exit near my office. This kind of location puts me in contact with many more potential patients from more than one suburb."

6. **Main thoroughfare.**
   Between a residential and business area, but make sure the noise doesn't interfere with your treatment of patients.

7. **Moderate traffic, pace, noise.**
    Make sure it has ample foot traffic. It is preferable to be on a street where the speed limit is 30 mph with many red lights on the corners.

8. **Corner locations.**
    People often need to stop at a light or stop sign and may notice your office sign. Also corner locations are easy to locate when visualizing directions — i.e. 10th and Pine is easier to picture than the middle of the block.

9. **Locate near a prominent location or landmark where people go regularly:**
    "Across from the post office, the library, the courthouse, south end of the mall."

10. **Convenient location such as just off a main artery or expressway.**
    Again, check if indoors area is quiet enough for your services. If you are downtown: Is public parking easily accessible and preferably free? Avoid being on a dead end street or cul-de-sac or on a one way street unless it is in a popular medical complex. Choose the side of the street, if possible, directed toward traffic returning from work. Be on a bus route. Is there a bus stop nearby, preferably outside your office?

11. **Good sign exposure.**
    Make sure that for the area you are in, you are allowed (via zoning regulations) good sign exposure. It should be sufficient size to be readable by any passing foot or auto traffic. Check the zoning regulations as far as a placement of a large sign — how close to the street it can be. If a large sign is not allowable on the building, can letters (and check how large) be painted on a window? Is a well lit sign permissible? Is the sign in proper proportion visibility-wise to other signs in the area? Does it communicate professionalism? Compliment the building? (Check with the landlord). Blend with the surroundings? Break the plane of people's vision (i.e. such as oblique angles)? Does it call attention? Is it tasteful and appropriate?

12. ***Neat, clean, well lit and appear to be busy enough to be well exposed and utilized.***
    In a shopping center in Port Hueneme, a large medical building was included in a rather large shopping complex with a 24 hour grocery store. As customers drive in 24 hours a day, they can't miss the large well lit oblique sign in tasteful letters advertising a ' Acupuncture Wellness Center.'

13. **Ground floor if possible.**

    If not, make sure there is an elevator. Sick people find it hard and less safe to climb a flight of stairs. (Consider your liability and insurance, as well). Ground floor practices are more visible.

14. **Place where you can have good marketing and education exposure.**

    In a shopping center, one acupuncturist tastefully used a slide presentation in her window to educate people to the advantages of acupuncture and the type of treatment performed in her office. This was very successful. This could be done with video equipment as well as with a vista viewer with an automatic on-off timer. Practices in shopping centers often put up a banner for exposure when they open: "New Acupuncture Office Now Open." It is quite effective. You must get permission from the shopping center management to do this. Make sure it is legal in your area.

15. **Make sure your location is a safe area where crime rate statistics are low.**

    Do you have adequate liability, fire, and police protection? Do you have dead bolt locks and insurance at a reasonable rate because of your location?

16. **Affordable Location.**

    Keep your costs down and overhead in control. Also, make sure the terms of your lease protect you financially (see lease agreements). Check with your local commercial real estate agents as to the going square footage rates in the area for office space to make sure you are paying a fair rate, as well as whether it fits within your budget. See if it fits to stretch to be where you want to be: to put up extra cash for quality locale and that you can make the necessary improvements within the time frame you need to start practicing.

17. **Good Layout.** (Refer to questionnaire and upcoming section on office layout.)

A number of these points were cited from Dr. Peter Fernandez's book, _How to Start a Profitable Practice from Scratch_, 1980, and the SBA pamphlet, "_Starting and Managing a Small Business of Your Own._"

Will the Office Meet Your Needs?

Below are some questions to ask yourself and others before deciding on office space. Answer these questions and go back and evaluate them afterwards with an overall + or --. Ideally you should have "yes" answers and "pluses". Look at your "minuses" and weigh them carefully against the pluses. See what you can do to eliminate as many negative answers as possible before you sign anything.

LOCATION, LOCATION, LOCATION!

+ - 1.   Will: ❑ the patient come to your place of business ❑ you go to their home ❑ both.

+ - 2.   Is the area you are practicing in zoned for your service? ❑ Yes ❑ No

+ - 3.   Is it a space where there is a demand for your services? (Survey!) ❑ Yes ❑ No

+ - 4.   How accessible, convenient, and desirable is your location for the clientele you want to appeal to? ❑ Poor ❑ Average ❑ Good ❑ Excellent

+ - 5.   Is it available to you or to a sublessee: ❑ 24 hours a day ❑ restricted

+ - 6.   Does your building or office space fit the criteria for an ideal locale? (Check previous pages on locale.) ❑ Yes ❑ No

+ - 7.   If you choose a remote location, will the savings of rent and personal pleasure offset 1) the reduction of business due to an inconvenient or low population area location and 2) the cost of advertising to make your services known? ❑ Yes ❑ No

THE OFFICE SPACE AND LAYOUT:

+ - 1.   How much square footage of floor space do you need?_____

+ - 2   Does this space have it? ❑ Yes ❑ No How much is it short?
_____ How much is it over? _____

+ - 3.   Can you rent out the extra space? ❑ Yes ❑ No Would you want
to do this? ❑ Yes ❑ No

+ - 4.   Are there enough rooms to accommodate your needs? ❑ Yes ❑
No

+ - 5.   Are the rooms spacious enough? ❑ Yes ❑ No

+ - 6.   Is the ceiling height sufficient? ❑ Yes ❑ No

+ - 7.   Are the entrances, exits, rest rooms, adequately laid out and up
to code? ❑ Yes ❑ No

+ - 8.   Is the front office partitioned or a separated room from the
reception area so that receiving area is relaxed and quiet? ❑ Yes
❑ No

+ - 9.   Is the front office partitioned so that financial business with
patients is handled from inside the business office, rather than
from the reception room? ❑ Yes ❑ No

+ - 10. If not, can the space be easily remodeled and cost-effective to
accommodate this? ❑ Yes ❑ No

+ - 11. Does the space have the capacity to handle expected patient
volume? ❑ Yes ❑ No

+ - 12. Does the space have the floor load you need for equipment?
❑ Yes ❑ No

+ - 13. Does the space meet your requirements legally? ❑ Yes ❑ No

+ - 14. Does the layout and floor plan meet your needs? ❑ Yes ❑ No

+ - 15. Could activities flow easily with it? ❑ Yes ❑ No

+ - 16. Can you expand later? ❑ Yes ❑ No

+ - 17. Are the adjacent tenants in the general complex compatible and
preferable? ❑ Yes ❑ No

+ - 18.   If you choose an upstairs office, is there an elevator? ☐ Yes ☐ No

+ - 19.   Is your office sign such that it can be easily seen from the street?
☐ Yes ☐ No

+ - 20.   If not, is it easy to find your office from within the complex?
☐ Yes ☐ No

+ - 21.   Is parking for patients: ☐ easily available   ☐ an adequate number of spaces ☐ non-pay or ☐ pay parking paid by you or your patients?

+ - 22.   Does the layout lend itself to adequate security? ☐ Yes ☐ No

+ - 23.   Is additional security provided? ☐ Yes ☐ No ☐ By landlord ☐ By you ☐ at landlord's expense ☐ at your additional expense.

+ - 24.   Will crime insurance be needed and available at a reasonable expense? ☐ Yes ☐ No

+ - 25.   Does it have enough space to rent to other practitioners to help subsidize your rent? ☐ Yes ☐ No

+ - 26.   Would it suit your needs if you needed to phase out renters and expand? ☐ Yes ☐ No

CONDITION OF THE OFFICE:

+ - 1.   Is the condition of the building and office: ☐ poor ☐ average ☐ good ☐ attractive ☐ architecturally pleasing

+ - 2.   Does it need: ☐ painting ☐ plumbing, electrical, and other maintenance repairs ☐ nicer landscaping ☐ updating ☐ upgrading ☐ added fire and crime protection devices.

+ - 3.   Is the electrical capacity adequate for your needs? ☐ Yes ☐ No

+ - 4.   Do you have enough telephone outlets? ☐ Yes ☐ No

+ - 5.   Does it have adequate or additional features which you need such as: ☐ natural and artificial lighting ☐ heating ☐ ventilation ☐ air-conditioning ☐ insulation for noise and smells (such as for moxa) ☐ music system

+ - 6. Will the landlord allow you to improve? ❑ Yes ❑ No ❑ At his cost ❑ At your cost ❑ With a tenant improvement allowance ❑ With the landlord's written approval.

+ - 7. Will janitorial services, gardening services, maintenance costs be provided ❑ by the landlord ❑ by you ❑ at landlord's expense ❑ at your additional expense.

FINANCIAL CONSIDERATIONS AND LENGTH OF OCCUPANCY:

+ - 1. Do you know the current market base office rents for the locations you are considering? ❑ Yes ❑ No

+ - 2. Is the office you are considering consistent with the usual rents? ❑ Yes ❑ No

+ - 3. Considering what you would pay for rent now and projecting rent increases, does this office warrant the cost you would pay for the annual cost of living rent adjustment in subsequent years? ❑ Yes ❑ No

+ - 4. Can you afford to rent alone? ❑ Yes ❑ No

+ - 5. If not, will you make provisions to rent to others? Comment:

_____

+ - 6. In addition to base rent for your square footage, do you pay a pro-rata share of the building's taxes, insurance, and maintenance? ❑ Yes ❑ No How much?_____

+ - 7. How much additional do you pay for utilities, liability insurance, and janitorial expenses? _____

+ - 8. How much would it cost you to remodel and furnish this office?

_____

+ - 9. Is your future occupancy guaranteed secure enough to warrant the cost and energy you would put into this office space? ❑ Yes ❑ No

+ - 10. Is the office space you want what you can afford? ❑ Yes ❑ No

+ - 11. If not, could the space be immediately made affordable? ❑ Yes ❑ No ❑ Maybe

+ - 12. If you are borrowing money to start your practice or remodel, will the lending institution approve a loan for this particular office in their package loan to you? ❑ Yes ❑ No

+ - 13. Can the cost be negotiated: ❑ by reduction in services provided by the landlord ❑ negotiating the terms of payment ❑ subletting space which is additional or after your normal hours ❑ other

+ - 14. Are the terms of your lease, rental, or purchase clear and checked by a lawyer? ❑ Yes ❑ No

+ - 15. Do you have a protected consecutive renewal option? ❑ Yes ❑ No

+ - 16. What are the consequences in the event that the building is sold?

+ - 17. Are you well-protected if problems occur with your arrangements? ❑ Yes ❑ No

(See Checklist for Leasing Office Space)

Checklist for Leasing Office Space

FINANCIAL CONSIDERATIONS:

Address of Lease:_____

$ sq. ft.____ Monthly payment $_____Yearly Payment $_____

DOES LEASE INCLUDE? (Yes answers are preferred)

+ - 1. Electricity   ❑ Yes ❑ No

+ - 2. Heating and cooling (gas, oil, or steam) ❑ Yes ❑ No

+ - 3. Parking facilities   ❑ Yes ❑ No

+ - 4. Janitorial service   ❑ Yes ❑ No

+ - 5. Snow removal (if applicable)   ❑ Yes ❑ No

+ - 6. Music system   ❑ Yes ❑ No

+ - 7. Accessibility 24 hour a day   ❑ Yes ❑ No

LENGTH OF LEASE:

(Example Questions: What are the consequences for you of obtaining 1 year with option for renewal? What is the business risk for you of obtaining a long 5-10 year lease? (ibid).

___1 year ___2 year ___3 year ___4 year ___5 year ____ Other

CONSTRUCTION:

+ - 1. Does outside of building need painting, landscaping, etc.? ❑ Yes ❑ No

+ - 2. Will landlord refurbish outside of building?   ❑ Yes ❑ No

+ - 3. Are there any sign restrictions, i.e. lighted sign, size of sign, etc.?
     ❑ Yes ❑ No

WILL LANDLORD PAY FOR INTERIOR REMODELING?

+ - 1. At no increase in lease payment? ❑ Yes ❑ No

+ - 2. At increase in lease payments.   ❑ Yes ❑ No
     If so, how much additional per month $____

+ - 3. To be paid by the practitioner in lump sum payment. ❑ Yes ❑ No

+ -   How much $_____

+ - 4. Will practitioner be responsible for interior remodeling? ❑ Yes ❑ No

+ - 5. Will practitioner receive a reduction in lease payments because he is renovating the landlord's property? ❑ Yes ❑ No

+ - 6. Does the practitioner have a "right of inspection" of the renovation provided by the landlord? ❑ Yes ❑ No

CLAUSES (~red)

+ - 1. Is the prac ... ts prior to completion of rer

+ - 2. Is the pr ... original condition
when he

+ - 3. Are de ... ow much $____

CLA(

+ - 1. If a d/ ... e practitioner interest
on h ... interest rate?____%

+ - 2. Do ... iew lease for a specific
tir

+ - 3. Γ ... blet" clause? ❑ Yes ❑ No

+ - 4. ... ate" clause, allowing the
... event the building becomes

+ - 5. ... assure low monthly payments
... el" for the lessee? ❑ Yes ❑ No

+ - 6 ... disability, or military service"
... cancel the lease in the event of
... ❑ No

+ - 7. ... right to remove his/her fixtures
... on of the lease? ❑ Yes ❑ No

+ - 8. ... iuse that states in the event of an
... will still be valid? ❑ Yes ❑ No

+ 9. ... uate liability, fire etc., insurance; if not,
... ❑ Yes ❑ No

10. ... ompetition" clause in it that prevents the
... ce to another (ibid.) acupuncturist? ❑ Yes
... No

... reprinted from Dr. Peter Fernandez, *How to Start*
... nd Ed. 1980.

Planning Your Office Space, Layout and Image

A health practice generally has the following minimal requirements: a consulting room, a business and reception area, a toilet and a treatment room/dressing room combination, and a storage area. You want the layout to be easy enough for you to function, room enough for expansion or adaption, and comfortable and appealing to your patients.

To assist you to create more of the practice you want, we have created space here for you to plan what image you want patients to see about you.
In planning you can use the cost sheets from the inventory section to cost out different items. We have made it as easy for you as possible to do this.

Planning office space includes planning the costs of remodeling, painting, carpeting, furniture, equipment, and supplies. It will also include those items which create your image. Estimate the costs that you must incur now, and what you plan to handle over time. Notice in the estimating section we have divided the estimating sheets into basics and an extension list of items. Image builders are also listed. For your convenience in planning your office space, we have divided the items to be estimated by room so you can consider in which rooms you want your biggest investments to go. Consider use of space, most useful items, comfort, pleasing appearance, cost effectiveness, and importantly, the attitude the image conveys.

Planning can be fun. Think about how you can cost effectively create or recreate the atmosphere that will attract and providing a healing atmosphere for your patients-- room by room. Describe the details, colors textures, educational aids or items you will use, smells you will emphasize, lighting details. What floor plan of furniture will invite a good feeling about you, promote you, and even promote interaction between your patients about your services. What will you create or add?

The Reception Room

Consultation Room

If you are considering having a consultation room, or a combined consultation/treating room: a neat desk, diplomas, display bookcase of acupuncture books, human models, pictures which promote your expression--all give the eye backup information which can add credibility and authority to your practice. What will you create or add?

_____
_____
_____
_____

Treating Room

Patients spend waiting time, preparation time, and time in the treating room when you are not present, as well as when you are. What room colors, focal pictures, smells, sounds, will help your patients relax? What displays, information, and equipment will you use to inspires confidence in your training, experience, and methods? What safe practice items will you use? Paper gowns? Clean and neatly pressed cloth gowns? Sterilization equipment and sanitary disposal means? Fresh paper on the treating table? Fresh sheets or covers?

_____
_____
_____
_____

Office

The location of the receptionist's desk, office or alcove should be:
1. Adjacent to a reception room with sufficient opening to view all reception room activities but private enough for phone calls
2. Adjacent to a hall or with some arrangement of semi-privacy for collections
3. Adjacent to the acupuncturist's consultation or treatment rooms.

The receptionist's desk area should be large enough to accommodate the following: your telephone system and answering phone, appointment book, daily accounting sheets, ledger tray with ledgers, treatment cards in tray and/or a computer or typewriter. Receptionist desks are often built in the shape of an L to accommodate these uses. Many reception areas are built to accommodate a counter at a higher level than the desk to allow patients a place to handle paperwork at the same time as the receptionist does.

The amount of space you as an assistant will need to function well is a minimum of 100 square feet and an additional 60 square feet for a second assistant. A number of front offices have a partitioned space in the front office where insurance is handled. Notice how other offices are set up.

A key, of course, is to work with the space you have, find ways to expand it by moving furniture, partitions, utilizing closets, wall racks ,etc. Be creative. If you have less than the above mentioned, ask the following questions and see if you can come up with some creative solutions to the use of your space:

- Can you use partitions to give privacy? Can you extend your space?
- Is the desk(s) in the best location to most effectively handle the needs of the office?
- Where can you use wall racks?
- Where can you add shelving?
- Where can you add file cabinets?
- What can be moved out of the front office and into a storage area or closet?
- What can be hung from the ceiling?
- Where can desk space be extended?
- Where can chairs be placed for easier function?
- Do the chairs roll easily from one place in the office to another?
- Where is the best place for relaying messages?
- Are you using a rack to store your files pulled in order for the day?
- Where is the best place for files which are pulled for the day?
- What additional nearby space could be utilized for storage of supplies, etc.?
- Is there a large (preferably lateral) filing cabinet which has a pull down enclosure in the front office area? Is it in the easiest place to access files?
- Are you using the "In and Out" file trays and message center in the best place to unclutter the desk?
- Do you have a file drawer or rack for your most often used forms and new patient packets?
- Do you need to add space to incorporate proper business machines, such as a photocopier, computer, typewriter?

Your Front Office Desk Area

_____

_____

_____

How To Set Up Excellent Telephone Communications

When you set up your office, you will need to install your telephone communications system. How you set up your telephone communications system can determine **more** than your degree of ease and privacy regarding your communications or availability for emergencies. The following are technical preparations, good solid reasons for use, and protocol for telephone use.

Technical Preparations

1. *Number of phones and lines.* There should be at least two to three telephones with multiple lines, preferably a rotary system, with a "hold" button in your office: One for the front reception desk, one for the insurance desk, and one for the acupuncturist's office. This allows for both incoming and outgoing calls to occur simultaneously by the staff, as well as one line for private calls by the acupuncturist. This is important if you want to:

   - be available at all times for patients to call in to make appointments.
   - be able to motivate a casual caller to make an office appointment.
   - be able to make outgoing calls to recall patients to reschedule,
   - be able to do outgoing calls to handle phone collections, or insurance without the reception room hearing.
   - be able to connect the acupuncturist for private conversations with other health providers and confidential telephone conversations with patients.

2. If you have an office-home telephone combination, illicit your family's cooperation in handling calls. Again, use more than one line.

3. If you use an *unlisted number*, always use it for outgoing calls.

4. Avoid annoying busy signals by limiting personal conversations, and using rotary lines.

Pager

This is valuable because you can leave a message on your answering machine to use the pager number for emergencies.

Answering machines vs. Paying for an Answering Service

With an answering machine:

■ You can program the exact message.

■ A machine doesn't make mistakes with phone numbers or names.

■ Price varies from just over $100 up to $400. After the initial investment for the machine, there's no additional cost. It's less than one year of an answering service's fee.

■ You can buy them with or without a voice activator. Machines are now being made to program the exact time of the message call, as well as if you dial a code number, you can call in for your message and it will play back the recorded message for you over the phone. Panasonic, Sanyo, Record-0-Call, phone mate, and code-a-phone are some of your best options.

■ Answering machines will answer within 1-5 rings on "immediate" or "delay."

■ If you don't want to record a message each day, you can make prerecorded message tapes for lunch/after hours/ special hours/ emergencies/and the weekend which play automatically when the machine is turned on.

The advantages of an answering service:

■ It's still considered more professional.

■ Machines are newer and not everyone is used to the idea of talking to a machine.

■ Not everyone is used to the idea of talking to a machine.

■ Services will cross-connect from your office to your home or call you in emergencies; machines can only take messages.

■ Human contact. People leave messages with people more than with machines.

Weigh these advantages and disadvantages carefully in making your decisions for phone setup and use.

FEES

How to Set Successful Fees

What Makes the Fee Standard You Set Successful?

- Value given, Value Received
- The competitive marketplace—what is usual, customary, and reasonable.
- Fees commensurate with treatment.
- Manner of communication in handling telephone and office procedures.
- Proper fee slip procedure and value of your services.[1]
- Manner of communication in Collection Procedures.[1]
- Workable financial plans, discounts, and allowances.[2]
- Establishment of consistent fees.

1. **Value Given, Value received.**

   As we have discussed earlier, patients must <u>perceive</u> that they receive full value for their services. It's your job and your assistant's job to communicate this. Do you communicate a sense of full value given in the time spent with the patient? Can the patient sense 1) the need for the visit 2) any change in his/her condition and 3) a clear workable direction given as a result of the services rendered? 4) Does the patient feel you are fully present with him or her? Communicating to patients the "extras" is a way of reinforcing their feeling of value. Understanding, compassion, education the extra time for explanation of care, procedures, and helpful equipment and product aids; comfortable surroundings; timely treatments; encouragement and reinforcement in following through on recommendations; reevaluating progress; and successful results all add value to the patient's experience of you and your practice. These are all built into the success of your fee.

2. **The competitive marketplace.**

   This means knowing the cost of like services in the marketplace. It is important to be aware of this because patients, as well as insurance companies, look at and are normally willing to pay according to the "usual and customary" rates paid in the area. It is acceptable and

---

[1]   Note section on "Income Generating Factors."
[2]   Note section on "Setting Financial Policies."

permissible to call a number of practitioners in the area in which you want to practice to survey what their fee schedule is for their services. Don't limit your calls to practitioners within your specified field. You may want to call treatment centers which handle specific conditions. See the "Fee Survey" with instructions for use in this section of the book. When you or your assistant call to find out this information, let them know you are looking for what is "usual, customary, and reasonable" for specific conditions in the community. Usually, other health practitioners are willing to help you and/or your staff as a service within the health profession. Remember, they were once starting out. Your call reminds them how they have had the same types of situations to handle.

The following basis for payment is defined as:

Usual: That fee ordinarily charged for a given service by an individual practitioner to his patient (i.e., his or her usual fee).

Customary: That fee that is within the range of fees usually charged by practitioners of similar training and experience for the same service within the same specific geographical area. In other words, this is a community fee.

Reasonable: That fee determined by responsible medical review authorities where medical circumstances of certain cases are unusual.

Insurance companies set usual and customary dollar amounts payable by them for treatments. You or your assistant can send in your charges to the insurance companies, and they will let you know if you are under or over their maximums dollar amounts for services rendered. The maximum dollar amounts, however, may be further defined by the policies purchased by the individual patient. Workers' Compensation publishes a fee schedule January 1 of each year which you can obtain by writing to your local Workers' Compensation Board. Again, use this only as a guide for the fees currently prevailing. Their standard is generally lower than the one set by most insurance companies. Take into consideration your costs to run your practice, as well as the quality and level of services you offer.

Be aware that insurance companies statistically set rates at which they will pay usual and customary charges prevailing in different areas. These rates are updated periodically. Price fixing by insurance companies for health care payment is illegal. Within the insurance companies are review committees to determine if "reasonableness" can be established to cover additional and warranted charges. Most insurance companies (or patients) will acknowledge what the practitioner charges as long as 1) the charge is consistent to all patients and 2) charges and required reports are presented clearly.

What is the impact of knowing the cost for treatment in the community? You don't run the risk of lowering the standard set in the profession which will affect insurance company standards of payment to professionals and patients. Secondly, the cost comparison shopper who calls the office can be set at ease when the receptionist tells the potential patient that the fee is fair and within usual and customary standards for a specific condition or general conditions. This allows the conversation to focus and shift to the quality of the practitioner and the quality of the treatment offered for the patient's benefit.

3. **Fees should be commensurate with treatment.**
    Insurance companies look at whether the fee is usual, customary and reasonable in the current market place for similar diagnoses. It is true that they also look at what acupuncturists charge in general as a flat fee. Because fees are often justified by diagnosis, try grading your fee by diagnosis. Cost of treatment takes into consideration primarily the complexity of the case; whether it is an initial, follow-up or reevaluation visit; type of procedures used; and the amount of time the service was rendered; and, of course, comparable cost in the marketplace not just for acupuncture, but of treatment results for specific conditions.

    Whether you code your services as brief, limited, intermediate comprehensive, or unusually complex, you will also need to consider if you should 1) charge for extended time or 2) reduce the fee for your treatment on that visit.

    Remember: In setting fees, most patients are not normally looking for a "cheap" or "the cheapest" practitioner. They are looking for the best one to assist them to health. Charging less than other practitioners to attract more patients puts your focus and the patient's attention more on the cost of what you offer than on the quality of what you offer. Be the best practitioner and charge accordingly. Establish consistency in fees.

4. **Establishment of consistent fees.**

   Patients and insurance companies want to know that your fees are established and consistent and will be so for the year. There may be occasions where you will need to raise your fees. Do this review of fees on a yearly basis. Analyze the cost of living index and how much your supplies and business costs to you have increased. Look at your goals and decide what would be appropriate in raising your fees. If you choose to discount, make sure you record this correctly. There are two primary ways you can discount:

   1. If you choose to offer less services than a code would normally cover, use a modifier (-52) to indicate reduced services. Many insurance companies will unquestionably cover these charges.

   2. If you choose to discount for senior citizens rates, give cash discounts or special family plan rates. Record your normal standard individual fees on your bookkeeping records. All fees need to be recorded as *"standard."* But you may adjust off any amount that is appropriate in the *"adjustment column"* on your ledgers—to the benefit of your patients. Make sure this is recorded through onto your day sheets.

How to Weigh Your Fees

1. Consider who and what services you will charge; how the socioeconomic location will affect your fee; how any incentive and reduced fee services will affect your fee and your referral base; and the way your practice will service patients.

    Focus on the value of your quality services. Make your first visit fee attractive so patients will come. Don't over do it on reduced fee services. The small leaks such as these in your financial base can create cash flow problems. Consider the section on "ways to expand patient payment" before you setup reduced fees. If you become popular because of your reduced fees, more than because of your services, emphasis will be built around low fee with high volume, and the "extras" in your practice are likely to diminish. You will need to choose between a quality increasing practice or quantity basic service practice when setting your fees.

2. Gather your factors of comparable value regarding achievable results obtained within the medical profession in your area of choice.

    In other words: What do other practitioners charge for achievable results? What amount of time does it take generally for them to see results with specific diagnoses? Use the "Fee Survey" and the diagnostic chart.

3. Get a sense of the value **you** give in treating a diagnostic grouping.

    Note the results you most often see. Although you can figures 1) a conversion factor (the dollar value you place on your time for services you perform) and 2) a unit of time value for each of the procedures you provide within the given diagnostic groups, you can 3) simply discern the value to put on your services through the following means:

4. The ultimate decision comes down to asking within, "What is the correct dollar amount to charge for this service?" Write it down.

5. "Is your answer clear?"
    A method I have seen used is the following:
    Tell yourself you would like a yes or no answer. This could be by a nod or shaking your head from side to side. If you get "yes," stay with it.

If you get a "no", ask "Are there any blocks? Is the number fair? Do I feel deserving? What is the new number? Is that clear?

6.   "Is that number in balance?"
What amount is charged must be in balance to both meet the market needs as well as meet your practice cash flow.

Hold your hands palm up in front of you. Use your hands like a balance scale. Put your answer to question #3 in one hand. If you are asking about the correct number for your services, test it against numbers which are higher or lower than your fist number by putting your second number in the other hand. Which answer feels lighter and clearer? Release the number or answer in the heavier hand. Ask, regarding the answer in the hand that feels lighter: "Does this answer feel in balance for me in my practice/my life?"

We all receive the answers to questions (such as the above) through different senses. Regarding the question of the correct amount to charge for a specific service, notice how some answers come in the form of vision. We see ourselves receiving X amount for a specific service. Some answers come in an auditory form. We hear a specific number in our mind. Some answers come kinesthetically--we feel a specific number is the correct one for us.

Whatever fees you set, it will either assist the profession of acupuncture in upgrading its standards or lower its standards by the fees you set. Insurance companies do look at over all fees charged within the profession in the geographical area.

Each year evaluate your fee structure with current trends in the profession and in your geographical area, your sense of value, and your results. Update your fee schedule. Do what fits for you within the context of the highest good of all.

You will be ready to do a final draft of your fee schedule after you have weighed your factors. The amount of your fees is an important decision, so take one step at a time. It will clarify as you follow the process.

Fee Setting: Answers About Charging

1. Consultations.

Most medical practitioners charge for their initial consultations. Usually in their following-up consultations specific recommendations are made. A mini-exam may accompany the examination as well. Often a report is written by the medical practitioner accompanying the consultation and this may be included in the cost of the consultation.

Some allied practitioners do not charge for a brief consultation. These consultations are used to build acceptance, educate the patient and allay any fears or considerations towards treatment. It is also used to find out if the patient's condition can be treated by acupuncture care.

A brief consultation is usually scheduled for approximately 15 minutes. The patient should be made aware of the time allowed and being told that he/she is welcome to come in 20-30 minutes early to fill out a history form which will assist the acupuncturist in determining if their particular approach would be appropriate for the patient. (Read the "Pre-consultation Dialogue" in Volume IV.)

If the nature of the consultation becomes more of an extended verbal examination, do consider this in your level of examination charge.

Follow-up consultations, either with another physician or practitioner, would usually be charged because of the nature of the consultation. Second opinions solicited by you and charged for by the other practitioner to you or directly to the patient should be made clear to those concerned beforehand. The patient will want to know if he/she will be responsible for these charges. If you charge a flat rate for a series of treatments and consultations are included, the patient should be aware of this.

2. Examinations.

(Use varying levels of services for your examinations).
This allows for flexibility and lower cost to healthier patients who require less examination and testing. This is not only ethical, but it also prevents the practitioner from becoming stereotyped by conducting only one type of examination. The practitioner can usually ascertain from the history given by the patient how much he or she will

need to do for the basic entrance examination. The healthy looking patient with little history of illness and rather acute sounding symptoms would have a simpler exam than a patient who is in considerable pain and is apparently more chronic. The patient who comes in with 1) pain and musculoskeletal complaints, 2) chronic organic ailments, 3) who is obviously very ill, and 4) one or more systems is quite run down—would involve a more comprehensive examination. Children usually will require a simple entrance exam. Have a specific fee for children exams and treatment.

Note the levels of service, definitions, and coding of services to see what fits. (See Volume II.)

Decide if you will do a consultation and examination on the first visit and whether you will treat that day. If you treat, under what circumstances? How much time will you spend for the level of complexity of examination and how much will you charge? What will you charge additionally if you treat? How will you code this?

3. **Report of findings (oral and/or written) and reevaluations.** *(1998 CPT code 99214.*
   Usually on the second visit an analysis of the physical examination and recommendations are made to the patient. (These recommendations can be written so the patient can visualize them, take them home, and work with them. (See recommendation sheets in the *Big Forms Packet.*) Allow 15-20 minutes for the evaluation. A copy of these recommendations can be sent also to the insurance company so they will cover the charges of this code. If the patient bills, this can be included with his billing and claim form. Reevaluations are vital and should be done usually anywhere between the fifth and tenth visit, according to the practitioner's discretion. This is so that the patient has a clear idea of 1) the progress he/she is making and 2) what further treatment and program should be continued. Do charge for these services. They involve extra work for you and your staff. These sessions are invaluable and build your practice. Any handouts you give your patients will many times be shown to others and "advertise" you and your services. The written reports given the patient also may establish an agreement of mutual responsibility. If these reports are used correctly, they can serve you in preventing malpractice.

4. Treatment.

Make sure your patients are aware of what the treatment entails ahead of time. This preparation will result in greater response to healing. Providing a viable treatment and home health care program will establish your authority and their willingness to work with you. Give full value to your treatments and don't give them away free. If patients have been served well, they will thankfully offer remuneration in return. They will work with you or your staff in paying for your treatments in a manner that works for you as well for them.

Treating health practitioners. Treat practitioners in your specific field of endeavor cost-free as a courtesy. It also builds rapport within your profession. It gives you and other professionals the benefit of learning from their colleagues' approaches and techniques, as well as provides for their personal healing. You may want to offer a 10-20%: professional discount to health practitioners, who are not acupuncturists.

Treating patients with addictions. For patients with smoking, drug, alcohol, and eating disorder addictions, consider introducing the prepayment of services policy as part of their 'treatment program'. See "Wellness Program Agreement" in the *Big Forms Packet)*. I would not recommend this as your general policy to patients unless you exclusively handle addiction patients. If you introduce this policy, introduce it as "part of the treatment program" which the practitioner sets up with the patient at the time of the consultation/examination/or report of findings.

Treating friends. When friends are in the office, they are patients. Your role is different. You are the practitioner. Some practitioners prefer to allow friends a discount or accept assignment of benefits from the insurance company alone and waive the patient's share of payment. Some practitioners prefer to work out exchanges or trades with friends. In these cases, they should be handled very specifically by the front office person in regards to record keeping. The front office person would write down the specific verbal financial agreement the acupuncturist and friend has discussed on the initial session. The office staff member would confirm what the payment of fee or exchange is at the front desk before the patient leaves. This prevents any misunderstandings or ill-feelings from occurring later on. The arrangement would be reviewed as is appropriate.

Many practitioners simply keep a neutral attitude regarding payment of fees. They have an agreement that friends support one another personally and financially in business. Business arrangements are handled by the front office staff. The office charges the standard fee and the fee is paid by the patient/friend.

Treating the clergy. Some practitioners have an agreement to treat clergy 1) as a free service, 2) discount—50%, or 3) "accept assignment only" from the church's insurance and do not bill the individual clergy. These are all considerations you will need to decide upon.

Treating the poor. There are clinics specifically sponsored by the government, churches, and charitable organizations which treat the poor on a sliding fee scale or free of charge. You may decide that you will do a certain portion of your practice as "charitable work". It is easiest to decide on specific hours of a particular day of the month if you wish to do this in your clinic. Otherwise, you can get a reputation for being the "poor man's practitioner" and find yourself rescuing others at the cost of your own sense of balance, both emotionally and economically. Perhaps you want to practice your service in a free service clinic on a particular day of month and offer this service separate from your regular practice. One option is to refer poverty cases to a charity clinic, perhaps one in which you offer part-time services. Whether you refer or not, remember: The greatest gift when that person comes to you in your clinic or calls on the phone, is the gift of hope, encouragement, and compassion. It may save that person's life.

Community service. You may offer to do free physical screening for the community at which time you may recommend that a patient come to you for treatment. In these cases, you would not charge for the screening; however, you would charge your regular fee if they came into your office for treatment.

5. **Services requiring additional time.**
   Many practices either dismiss or are slack in regards to charges for additional time, along with well-deserved remuneration for additional services. Be specific in recording on the fee slips the code for additional time or modalities. Insurance companies do recognize additional time if the treatment program warrants. As mentioned earlier, if you do offer some extras at no charge, be sure these are

itemized on the patient's bill as extra time at N/C (no charge). This builds patient awareness of the "extras" you give which make you special.

6. **Disposable needles, supplements, herbs, nutritional adjuncts, supports, magnetic supports or jewelry, relaxation tapes.**

    Disposable needles are an expense to you and can be charged to the patient.

    Many practitioners are stocking products which support their patient follow-through with home recommendations. These products can be included in your standard treatment or charged as an adjunct to services. Most practitioners charge for these products because they are added income producers which not only support their home care instructions, but help stabilize cash flow in the practice.

    Most insurances will not cover vitamins and supplements. However, some insurance companies will cover supports. (Note specific procedure codes for supplements, orthopedic cushions and supports). It is important to receive payment at the time of service for these items since most companies will not cover these items.

    More and more practices are keeper larger inventories of health care products to supplement their patient needs and help stabilize that practice cash flow. Note the "Inventory of Supplies" within the "Total Practice Equipment and Supplies List" of the financial planning section.

7. **Tests.**
    Lab, urinalysis, hair analysis, blood work. Usually these are out of office charges. It is recommended the patients pay you directly if you are billed. Otherwise, patients can pay the other facility directly. These charges generally are paid for as rendered.

Fee Schedule Survey

You are looking for comparable value of achievable results obtained within the medical profession. When you or your assistant calls to find out the information below, let the office manager or practitioner know who you are and what your situation is. Ask: "Would you be willing to assist us regarding 10 questions we have on service codes and fees so that we can set our fees according to what is "usual, customary, and reasonable in the community" for specific conditions?". Also ask: "Is this time convenient?" Or, if it isn't, ask: "What time would be best to call you back Occasionally, you may find someone pressured or, for some reason, uncooperative. However, most other successful practitioners are reminded that they were once starting out and they have had the same types of situations to handle. Your call may also serve the other offices by reminding them, as well, to keep current with prevailing rates. Usually, other health practitioners are willing to help you and/or your staff as a service within the health profession.

Make several copies of this page as well as the Recording Fees page and make your comparison calls.

1. What is the cost of your treatment program for (name the type: weight-loss, smoking, etc.)?

2. What is your success rate?

3. What is the number of average visits or range of visits for specific conditions? (Name whichever ones you wish to specialize in or would be applicable to your practice)

4. Do you charge by the visit or by the program?

5. Do you see successful results in doing so?

6. What does your office charge for specific codes such as: (name)

7. How much time does the practitioner generally spend per visit with patients with (name specific conditions)?

8. Do you have a flat rate charge for returning patients? How much and what procedure code do you use?

9. How much time do you generally allow in the schedule per visit for established patients?

10. What does your office charge for the service coded examinations?

(See Current Year's Procedure Codes (included as a free supplement to the book) listed by code, procedure, level of complexity, and time.)

How to Determine Your Fees

One way to establish fees commensurate with treatment is to classify your fee by diagnosis. You can classify it according to:

1. Complexity.
2. The amount of time spent with the patient.
3. The number of estimated treatments required to achieve comparable or better results than is offered by other practitioners in the medical or allied medical field.
4. What cost is comparable in the marketplace for treating the specific diagnosis.

Break the cost of the treatment program down to a fee schedule by visit. The appropriate codes then can be assigned to fit the level of complexity of the visit.

On the next page we have included a fee schedule by a practitioner who has built an _outstanding_ reputation in the medical community. His excellent results warrant the fees he charges. He practices based on:

1) the value he feels he gives to the patients and the results he sees.
2) comparable value of achievable results obtained within the medical profession.
3) the socioeconomic climate of the area

While a beginning practitioner could not charge such fees, someone who is well known and respected in the larger medical community certainly can.

EXAMPLE OF A FEE SCHEDULE BY PROGRAM

Category A   Program of 10 Treatments: $1000 prepaid.

Category B   Program of 10 Treatments: $590 prepaid.

Category C   Program of 10 Treatments: $420 prepaid.

Category D   Program of 10 Treatments: $390 prepaid.

Category E   Program of 10 Treatments: $900 prepaid.

Category R   Program (unspecified; depends on type of condition and severity).

Category S   Program of 5 Treatments: $200 prepaid.

Category W   Program of 15 Treatments: $400 prepaid.

FEE SCHEDULE BY VISIT

Category A   The value of treatment would be $110 per session of 10.

Category B   The value of treatment would be $70 per session of 10. Initial visit is $70.

Category C   The value of treatment would be $45 per session of 10.

Category E   The value of treatment would be $100 per session of 10. Initial session is $200.

Category R   Depends on type of condition and severity.

Category S   Initial session would be at $100; subsequent at follow-up visit rate — $50 per session of 5 treatments.

Category W $35 for first 15 treatments; $30 following. $50 Initial; 25 visits @$25.

Problems in Category A are only to be treated by themselves. No additional ailments are specifically treated simultaneously. For other categories, additional ailments will be treated at $10 additional ailment per treatment. There will be an equipment usage fee of $10 additional for laser treatment. No needle treatment will be administered. Food supplements, herbs, and vitamins are not included in the fees.

Diagnostic Grouping for Determining Your Fees

This sample is used with the fee schedule on the previous page.

Diagnostic Group: Letter and Description

A Addictions to Alcohol, Drugs, Food, Smoking, Sugar, Withdrawal Syndrome, Frigidity, Impotence, Infertility, Premature ejaculation, Heart disorders .

B Age spots, Alopecia areata, Alzheimer's Disease, Angina pectoris, Anxiety, Backache, Baldness, Barre-Guillain Syndrome, Arrhythmia, Astigmatism, Breast enlargement, Bunions, Cataracts, Chest pains, Color blindness, Complexion problems, Cystitis, Depression, Diabetes, Disc herniated or ruptured Dupuytren's contracture, Dyspnea, Gallbladder disorders, Glaucoma, Growth, impaired, Gum disorders, Hair restoration, Hepatitis, Herpes, Immunological disorders, Intrastitial cystitis, Iritis, Irregular Heartrate, Jaw disorders, Joint disorders, Keratitis, Kidney Disorder, Lower back pain, Lupus, Macular Degeneration, Manic Depressive syndrome, Memory problems, Multiple Sclerosis, Muscle disorders, Myopia, Nervousness, Night blindness, Numbness, Body odors, Optic neuritis, Paralysis, Poor circulation, Premature aging, Prolapses of Rectum, Stomach, Uterus, Psoriasis, Retinal disorders, Reynold's disease, Scar tissues, Side effects of chemotherapy and/or drugs, Pruritis, Stress, Stye, TMJ syndrome, Loose teeth, Torn cartilage, Torn ligaments, Torn muscles, Urinary incontinence, Warts.

C Acne, Adrenal disorders, Allergies, Ankle problems, Anorexia, Arthritis in multiple joints, Bedwetting, Bell's palsy, Bone disorders, Bronchitis, Bursitis, Cancer pain, Circulation disorders, Colitis, Corns, Cough, Cramps, Deafness, Dermatitis, Diarrhea, Digestive disorders, Diverticulitis, Diverticulosis, Dyspepsia, Eczema, Edema, Elbow problems, Flatulence, Food allergies, Frequent urination, Gastritis, Gout, Gynecological disorders, Headache, Hearing loss, Hemorrhoids, Hiccups, High cholesterol, Hives, Hyperthyroidism, Hypoglycemia, Hypothyroidism, Indigestion, Insomnia, Intestinal disorders, Itching, Jaundice, Liver disorders, Menopausal syndrome, Menstrual disorders, Migraine headache, Nasal polyps, Nausea, Neck problems,

Neuralgia, Neurasthenia, Osteoporosis, Pain, all Types, Parkinson's disease, Periodontitis, Perspiration, excessive, Rash, Rheumatism, Rhinitis, Sciatica, Scoliosis, Shortness of breath, Shoulder problems, Sinus problems, Skin disorders, Smelling disorders, Sprains, Stiffness of joints, Stomach disorders, Strabismus, Strain injury, Sugar addiction, Tarsal tunnel syndrome, Taste disorders, Tendonitis, Tennis elbow, Tic douloureux, Tinnitus, Trigeminal neuralgia, Ulcers of legs or digestive tract, Urticaria, Varicose veins of legs or digestive tract, Vertigo, Walking problems, Wrist problems, Yeast Infection.

D Constipation, Facelift, Hiatal hernia, High blood pressure, Hyperactivity, Prostrate disorders, Common cold.

E Emotional Problems, Whip lash.

R Bladder disorders, Blood disorders, Eye disorders, Foot disorders.

S Smoking.

W Overweight, Weight control.

Fee Schedule Worksheet

Recommendation:

- Record fees by treatment program and by visit.
- Photocopy enough pages of this form to record your own fees, as well as comparable fees, or
- Make up your own form to fit your own needs.

- Make up an additional page based on the information you find for your area on the codes for Workers' Compensation companies, those insurance companies still RVS, and state aid. (Use procedure codes listed in the **Volume II** or in the ICDA-9-CM Code Book). You will also need to list both CPT and RVS codes for physical medicine modality and procedures with you fees by visit.

- Computing fees by unit value is used by workers' compensation primarily. Example: Comprehensive Exam = X units @ $ unit = $, ie.. Comprehensive Exam = 17.5 units x $6.15 = $107.63. This method is a more 'time oriented" method of determining fees.

EXAMPLE FEE SCHEDULE BY DIAGNOSIS
USING 1998 CPT CODING

Record fees by treatment program and by visit. Photocopy enough pages of this form to record your own fees, as well as comparable fees; or, make up your own form to fit your own needs.

DIAGNOSTIC GROUP	CODING CPT	DESCRIPTION	TREATMENT PROGRAM FEE PER X #OF SESSIONS	FEE PER SESSION ONLY
A	99205	Initial Comprehensive Exam/Hist.	___ ___	___
	99215	Comprehensive Follow-up	___ ___	___
B	99205-52	Comprehensive Exam/Hist.	___ ___	___
	99213	Level 3 Follow-up visit	___ ___	___
C	99203	Level 3 Exam/Hist.	___ ___	___
	99212	Level 2 Follow-up Visit	___ ___	___
D	99204	Level 4 Exam/Hist.	___ ___	___
	99214-52	Level 4 Follow-up Visit	___ ___	___
E	99244	Level 4 Comprehensive Consult.	___ ___	___
	99215	Level 5 Comprehensive Follow-up	___ ___	___
R		Depends on condition	___ ___	___
S	99205-52	Comprehensive Exam/Hist.	___ ___	___
	99212	Level 2 Follow-up Visit	___ ___	___
W	99203-52	Level 3 Exam/Hist.	___ ___	___
	99211	Brief Follow-up Visit	___ ___	___

CODED SERVICES
97780	Acupuncture one or more needles; without electrical stimulation
97781	Acupuncture one or more needles; with electrical stimulation
99070	Supplements, Supplies and Materials (50-100% markup)

Other: Make up an additional page based on the information you find for your area on the codes for Workers' Compensation companies, those insurance companies still RVS, and state aid. You will also need to list both CPT and RVS codes for physical medicine modality and procedures with your fees by visit.

Incentive and Reduced Fee Services

Cash paying discount for non-insurance patients:

Standard percentage payable per visit by insurance patients who "Assign Benefits" to the office:

Senior Discount:

Family Plan Discount:
    Second member:
    Child under 12:

Wellness Plan Monthly Rate:

Prepayment Discount for Treatment Programs
    (Non-addiction) or for "by Visit" services:

Trades you will use:
    Percentage of treatment you will allow for trade:

Other health practitioners (except other acupuncturists):

Clergy discount:

Poverty income level discount:

No charge services:
    Consultation--first 15 minutes/public relations or other:
    Specific days and hours you will donate on an appointment basis:
    Out of clinic services:
    Other acupuncturists:

    Your staff:

Discount as per individual agreement only:

Procedure Coding Your Services / Fees

When acupuncturists make up their fee schedules, superbills, or fee slips, the correct procedure codes should be printed on your forms. Most insurance companies require that you have a code for your services, and will reject claims with missing information on them—particularly procedure codes. The proper procedure codes are outlined in 1) the CPT code book and 2) the Workers' Compensation Fee Schedule, and 3) your state aid code guideline materials.

"The Physician's Current Procedural Code Terminology" is a code book of the types of services provided by practitioners and has been standardized for universal use. The CPT code book can be purchased by calling 1 (800) 621-8335 or writing to the AMA Department of Health Care Resources:

CPT Publications Order Dept.
P.O. Box 7046
Dover, DE 19903-7046

Acupuncturists also use the diagnostic code book, the most recent ICDA-( )-CM which can be purchased from the AMA. The AMA also carries the largest nationwide health insurance billing directory which lists all of the insurance companies and their 800 numbers to verify claims coverage. This "Insurance Directory" is put out by Medicode and is kept updated.

Procedure code books are updated as often as yearly. Levels of complexity of services are described, as well as modifiers of these standard codes. Many of the procedure codes, such as the "Office Visits" are the same for CPT and most RVS (relative value standard) coding. Special therapeutic services, physical medicine and acupuncture codes vary. At this writing, there was no specified CPT code for acupuncture. It has been considered a write-in: "unlisted medical, therapeutic or miscellaneous procedure or an addition to an office visit." "State aid" uses their own codes. Double check all codes before using them.

Workers' Compensation in most states is still functioning on the RVS (relative value standard) code as of this printing, as well as some insurance companies. The state is not subject to the Federal Trade Commission ruling that "price fixing is illegal". The Workers' Compensation Fee Schedule with the RVS codes and values can be obtained from your state Labor and Industrial Relations Board.

Know and use proper procedure codes. A rule of thumb in knowing which codes to use with your fee structure is to notice:

1) the description of the procedure.
2) the complexity of the condition.
3) the amount of time allotted.
4) the cost allowance where indicated.
5) type of case — Workers' Compensation or private patient.
6) which coding standard—CPT or RVS—is listed on the "Verification of Insurance Coverage Form" filled out by your patient.

If the CPT code is not available for your service, your options are:

■ 1. Write the type of office visit code with the word "acupuncture" after it.

■ 2. Use the unlisted procedure code and specify type of service.

■ 3. Use the RVS code for your state, for Workers' Compensation where indicated, and where specific insurance companies are on the RVS standard.

■ 4. Call the local AMA and ask them which codes are normally used for acupuncture and related therapies in your area at this time.

Some insurance companies will adapt the RVS codes to the CPT codes and conversely so that the claims can be paid. If not, you will need to recode your services and resubmit the claim. It is best to have your patients fill in the "verification of insurance coverage form" (which specifies CPT-RVS coding) before you mark the day's service code so payment for services is efficient and trouble-free. Mark either "CPT" or "RVS" on the top of the patient's financial ledger. When ledgers and fee slips are printed, put on both the CPT and RVS codes (double checked for your area). You or staff can then easily mark the day's codes.

Check yearly to update current coding. Acupuncture codes and fees are under review and may be further differentiated in the future. For example, there may be differentiation in acupuncture codes for laser acupuncture vs. needle acupuncture. Also depending upon the state in which you practice, acupuncture may be considered as a surgical code, a miscellaneous medical therapeutic service, or a physical medicine code. The classification may affect your status of payment, which is particularly so in workers' compensation cases. Acupuncture may also be classified under two headings in one state depending on whether it is for a workers' compensation case or not., Take note that even though acupuncturists may be licensed as an independent practitioner in a state, workers' compensation may require a physician referral to treat their cases, which affects the classification of acupuncture for fee status. The status of acupuncture will no doubt change in the future.

We have included the latest CPT coding available at this printing either in the appendix or as a supplement added to this book. Again, you must check the codes yearly against the procedure code books to make sure they are still accurate.

Note: As you look at the "Fee Schedule" a few pages prior, you will note there is a procedure code associated with the description of services. If there is a -52 this means that the fee reflects a reduced fee for services rendered. Not all of your fees for a particular code will be the same. A -52 is more likely to be paid upon by insurance companies than using a service code which is more limited and "adding" charges signified by a -22 on the end of the service code.

FINANCIAL SYSTEMS AND POLICIES

Evaluating and Setting Your Best Financial System

Look at the pluses and minuses and do what works best for you.

1. **CASH PRACTICE ONLY.**

   A cash practice often produces the highest percentage of collections in relation to services rendered, but it has the least growth potential. It keeps your "accounts receivables" relatively low as well as bad debts. It can limit income by keeping away patients who have insurance and who want to void the large outlay of cash. A cash practice can reduce the potential for more than one person per family from having the care they need at the same time.

2. **EASY CREDIT PRACTICE.**

   An easy credit practice can create the potential for the highest growth, but it tends to produce the greatest amount of "Accounts Receivable" and bad debts. Since overhead will always rise in relation to services rendered, credit that is too easy is highly undesirable. However, it does make it easier for patients to come to you.

3. **MODIFIED CREDIT PRACTICE.**

   By modifying credit you can combine the advantages of both a cash and easy credit practice. Simply require all patients to pay cash for the first visit. Have cash patients pay for each subsequent visit (or current monthly bal   ance); and have your insurance patients cover a percentage of each visit after their deductible has been met. Fifty percent coverage works very well. The range in many offices is between 20-50%. Most insurance policies cover 80%, but it is on customary and usual charges and usually does not include supplements, nutritional supplements, and many supplies.

Cash Payment Patients

As mentioned earlier, the biggest factor to remember is that patients usually do not go to a practitioner because he/she is "cheap" or the "cheapest". They go to a practitioner because he/she is the best and can assist them with wellness; and he/she is willing to do what it takes for this to occur. Set your financial fees and terms of payment in line with what fits what you offer and is appropriate for your area.

Pros and Cons of Sliding Fees

Payment of sliding fees are usually affected by the patient's value of the treatment and ability to pay, your value of the treatment, and their willingness to value your level of service. Notice how you "slide" on how you feel about and view your services. It will show: 1) in the way your policy is interpreted, 2) in the manner in which payments are asked for, and 3) in the timing, amount and attitude in which payments are made. The outline of advantages and disadvantages is as follows:

Advantages

■ This may allow more people to come to you who could or would not otherwise come to you or prolong their treatment care.

Disadvantages

■ There are disadvantages of an easy credit practice as listed previously.

■ It is difficult to predict any kind of cost control of 1) how much income you can expect, and 2) how much you can outlay in expenses. Sliding fee income fluctuates. Setting fees based on the value of treatment serves to stabilize income.

■ It can be a disadvantage when fees and payments are based more on the patient's value of the treatment and ability to pay than on your value of the treatment and their willingness to value your level of service.

■ It is costly in processing paperwork to establish and reestablish the basis of payment. How often would you evaluate when a patient's income changed and adjust when the fee would change? Is the patient going to want to assess his financial picture every month and will he want to choose to do accurate monthly financial statements to determine what his fee should be? This may be more of a burden on your patients than a help. (For low-income patients, who have state aid, these patients will need to prove their finances on a monthly basis. If you do accept state aid patients, have them photocopy the same records that they use for state aid.)

■ It generally is not cost effective to process this paperwork. Medi-Cal or Health Initiative in California, for example, allows for 2 visits per month among health care providers for treatment at a set charge. Is it worth processing their paperwork? Would you request that patients do their own state aid billing and pay you cash?

- It may tend to become a low-income patient practice. In that case, it could demand a lot more work on your part for income to increase and you risk an unstable return.

The next section provides an alternative to sliding fee scale based on patient income.

Forms of Payment during Practice Stages

In order to make it easier for patients to continue care, there are numerous alternatives to reducing fees. Consider the following:

Start up to stabilization phase of practice, particularly:
- Set up a Mastercard / Visa merchant account so patients can put their treatment on their credit card. This takes the pressure off both you and the patient to come up with cash. Setting up your merchant account is well worth the effort, and the charges per month are very minimal. Check a couple of banks for differences in monthly charges. Generally you will get your merchant account at a bank you have an account with already because you have established a credit rating with them. If you are looking for another bank to do business with, consider the ease of obtaining a merchant account when you first look for your bank. Mastercard and Visa take approximately 3% of the payment—an inexpensive service—in relationship to the cost of labor to do long and short term billing or calls and letters to keep up collections.

During stabilization to growth phase, particularly:
- Work out a long or short term payment plan with patients if needed. Don't
emphasize this approach. Use it as a viable option to quitting care prematurely. Still treat patients at a rate that you know your treatment is worth.

- Work out some options with the patient: Perhaps the patient can take out a loan for long term care, obtain insurance coverage, or apply for Mastercard or Visa and then put treatment charges on his/her card to be paid off at the patient's convenience.

- Have your patient write a postdated check for when he will be next paid.

- Work out a long or short term payment plan with patients if needed. Don't emphasize this approach. Use it as a viable option to quitting care prematurely. Still treat patients at a rate that you know your treatment is worth.

- Charge less for children than for adults. (They may take less time to treat.)

- Give a senior citizen discount. One option is to charge a base rate, but include more services; or, give them a set lower rate (10-20% lower than your usual rate).

Understand that discounting refers to time, services, and financial plans. Financial policies must be carefully built into your program, if you discount on a regular basis. It is wiser to create discounts more as bonuses and incentives for prompt and cash payment, rather than for primary services rendered. If you mix your heart with finances, you may find that in your desire to be kind, you often times give away your services and additional time. You may end of paying the price by developing a sloppy practice both in financial and time management, which in the end creates uncomfortableness and lack of clarity with your patients. In discounting, remember that services must be: usual, customary, and reasonable; be in line with creating balance in your practice; still serve to create full value for your time and services.

Form of Patient Payment

- **Cash and valid personal check.**
  This is the most preferable form.

- **Mastercard/Visa payment.**
  One of the easiest forms of receiving payment in full from the patient at the time of service. No billing of the patient is required and there is no payment plan involving a long drawn out wait for full payment. It is very clean.

- **Money order.**
  This is like receiving a personal check. There are no complications with money orders.

- **Travelers checks.**
  These need to be signed by the patient and signed over to the practitioner.

- **Post dated checks.**

Assure the patient you will not cash his or her postdated check until the date that it will clear. Do not put it through the office books until the date designated on the check. Earmark the check and the service fee slip with a yellow sticky stating: "Hold until _____(date)."

- **Payment plan checks.** (A series of post dated checks).
  These are being utilized increasingly by health practitioners because of the state of the economy, and it has statistically been proven to reduce collection problems—i.e., debts that otherwise would not be collected or simply written off. Set a maximum amount, for example, $100, which you will not go beyond, when extending credit. Also set a minimum amount that you will accept. Determine how many payments you will allow. Remember that this is a guide.

- **Trades.**
  This can be for office services such as typing, bookkeeping, window washing, landscaping, office cleaning, massage exchange, tickets to an event, cooked meals, services you need at home. Utilize any other exchangeable crafts. Keep a record of office visits and your usual fees. Let the patient keep a record of their services and value. Monthly evaluate the new balance financially.

Financial Policies Which Work

The major types of financial plans for building your practice, as well as for providing a workable fee structure are:

1. Cash Payment Policy
2. Payment Plan
3. Monthly Billing
4. Family Policy
5. Prepayment of Services
6. Workers' Compensation policy and liens
7. Personal injury policy and liens
8. Assignment of insurance policy

Individual cash plans. You set your basic cash rate based on the individual plan. This means your basic discount is for payment over the counter at the time of service. Because you do not have to fill out insurance forms, you can explain the patient you can pass the discount on to your cash paying patients. Will you offer a cash paying discount?

Insurance plans. The major allowance many practitioners offer insurance patients is what is called "assignment of benefits". This means the practitioner will allow the patient to authorize direct payment to him/ her from the patient's insurance company for that portion of the payment of fees which the insurance company would pay toward services. The practitioner may set any number of policies in this regard asking the patient for partial payment based on the amount of payment portion that the insurance would not normally pay. This may range from 20-50%—whatever the practitioner feels he/she needs to cover his/her operating costs and keep a good cash flow occurring.

Credit is usually extended for X amount of time in awaiting payment for services by the insurance company. It is wise to set a specific limit of time by which payment must be received by the insurance company or when the patient would then be responsible for payment. Some practitioners prefer to simply have the patient pay at the time of service, give the patient a superbill insurance statement, and have the patient receive a reimbursement from the insurance company.

Payment plans and monthly billing. These can be offered to individuals who do not have insurance (usually). The more options you can give your patients in working out how they will pay your standard fee, the more they will not see your standard fee as a barrier to treatment. I would not "promote" these two plans. I would promote cash paying over the counter. However, it is important to make sure the fee is a workable one. If cash or credit card over the counter becomes a problem, the workable thing is to offer the next viable option. Definitely do payment plans for accounts over $100.

Senior citizen discounts. These can be incentives to persons on Social Security and Medicare. You may want to merely not charge for an extra modality like TENS rather than discount your primary service.

Family plans. You may want to discount for succeeding members of the family, who would possibly hesitate to have the health care unless they had the discount. Family discounts encourage families to participate in health care. (See Family Plan in the *Big Forms Packet.*)

Wellness plans. These are what are know as maintenance care package plans. These are annual plans which are not for patients with acute or chronic conditions. These plans are also not for patients who expect their insurance to pay, because insurance only pays for sickness or accident related illness. A wellness plan is a cash plan where the patient pays for the initial exam and is on a 12 month program with X # of treatments at a specific rate per month. It includes wellness counseling sessions - X # at $XX. It may also include patient education tapes with X # of sessions (listening sessions) at $ XX/per month. All of the above may be included in one package price.

Trades. Allow for flexibility in the type of forms of payment.

Treatment programs. Treatment programs are offered to patients for the following advantages: (Communicate this information to the patient, if it fits.)

1. Overall fees are lower, which gives the patient an opportunity to save funds.
2. The fee is fixed so the patient can budget for his or her health needs.
3. Established programs build a sense of commitment to regularly and consistently take treatments. This enhances the results.
4. The program enables the staff to better plan treatments to enhance and monitor the patient's progress.
5. The program simplifies bookkeeping procedures, cuts office costs, and passes savings on to the patient.

Fees by program are prepaid unless other arrangements are made. These fees are discounted. Fee by visit can be offered at a standard rate per treatment type. Be aware that prepayment of fees may be illegal in certain states and have negative consequences. See "Financial Policies Which work" for further explanation of pros and cons.

Prepayment of services merits more consideration before implementing it, so we'll discuss it in greater depth here. A prepayment policy means that fees are payable for services in advance of the services being rendered. The payment would either be on the date of service or before a series of treatments are initiated, and one sum for all the services is paid. A prepayment policy is used primarily with treatment programs, rather than with payment on a visit by visit basis.

If you serve a wide range of health needs, I would not recommend this as a general policy. Most patients exhibit the degree of trust and responsibility warranting payment of services after services are rendered--as part of the returning cycle of value given for services. Therefore, it is not necessarily appropriate as a policy for most patients *unless* you exclusively handle addiction patients.

If you do use a prepayment policy for addiction patients or for those you see this policy would benefit, you would explain on the phone to these new patients that the prepayment of services *is part of* the treatment program. If you do not exclusively serve addiction patients, you would keep your general policy of "payment of services after services are rendered on the first visit." Communicate that this procedure establishes a number of benefits in addition to credit with your office. At the initial consultation or consultation-examination with the patient, the acupuncturist--not the office staff--can establish the prepayment plan as part of the treatment program. An agreement that has been used effectively is the "Wellness Program Agreement." How appropriate this will be for you depends on the type of addiction patients you serve and the way you set up your program for addiction patients.

Practices which would probably not use the wellness program agreement would be those who are supplemented or funded by a public service organization, and can afford to have a low cost or no cost financial policy with addiction patients. These practices generally incorporate counseling and are able to have a loose structure for addiction patients where financial obligations and controls are removed.

Prepayment of .services may serve you if the below considerations and communications are made.:

1. **Legal implications:** Check with your state medical board. In some states, prepayment of services may be illegal.

2. **Individual healing rate:** Before the patient agrees to prepay services, remind the patient that each individual heals at a different rate. X number of treatments does not imply cure. You don't want a patient to feel mislead by any promise, statement or implication that they will be healed at the end of the prepaid services. If you communicate to the patient the statistics of the results you have generally observed with certain procedures which would relate to his or her condition, inform the patient that the patient's response will be unique to him or her.

3. **Commitment to patient success.** Inform the patient at the beginning that you will do a reevaluation of their condition on the (whatever you see as appropriate) visit midway through the treatment series to assess their progress and direction. Healing may not be complete at the end of the prepaid services, and you would not want them to feel that they failed. Renegotiate the treatment series extension.

   If you do use the Patient Wellness Program Contract, have the patient read the agreement out loud to you and sign. Keep a copy with the chart or treatment record and give one copy to the patient. Record on the fee intercommunication slip to your staff the fact that this patient is on a prepayment plan. If the patient is willing to honor the above commitment, this is an indication that he or she is willing to work with you on clearing the addiction or problem. He or she is then considered to be a potentially successful patient. Thank the patient for his/her accountability and reinforce evidence of this.

4. **Clear communication of patient and acupuncturist responsibilities.** Tell the patient in your words that he/she is responsible for his or her own healing process. Remember, that you are the catalyst for their healing process. It is illegal to imply, promise, or state that you can cure the patient. Your home care recommendations will help support this premise.

5. **Ability of the patient to prepay and provide insurance which preauthorizes payment.**
   Prepayment of total services is more an option to those patients who have insurance. Many company insurances cover patients at least 80% and increasing numbers of policies will cover most health care services for addictions, such as for alcohol. Use your "Verification of Insurance Coverage Form (forms packets) to verify and get pre-authorization for payment from the insurance company.

These are the basics. *Volume II* covers procedures to carry out your financial plans and policies. The *Big Forms Packet* and the Insurance Forms Packet contain a number of forms to implement clear financial policies and procedures.

Selecting Your Own Financial Policy

Every office has a financial policy, whether it is written or stated. Developed below are a list of questions to consider in building or clarifying your office policy.

After you have considered your financial policy, get clear in your office first what you communicate "as a team" to your patients. Patients need to feel some consistency in your approach. Staff need to be in agreement on what they communicate to patients. If they are not in agreement and clear on this point, it may cause some resentment between one another, as well as among the patients.

Policy Building Questions

❑ 1. Will you have a written financial policy ❑ for patients or ❑ for staff only?

❑ 2. Will you post your fees ❑ for patients or ❑ for staff only?

❑ 3. How often will you update your financial policy? In the beginning it will require careful setting and review, but normally ❑ every 6 months ❑ yearly ❑ as statistics and circumstances warrant. How often will you update your fees? ❑ every 6 months ❑ yearly ❑ as warranted. How will you communicate this to your patients? ❑ verbally by front office staff ❑ posted fee schedule ❑ for staff ❑ for patients ❑ patient letter

❑ 4. Who is in charge of handling financial policy questions? ❑ you ❑ office manager ❑ both of you together

❑ 5. Who has the authority to approve financial plans and arrangements? ❑ your office manager ❑ both of you together ❑ other

❑ 6. What payment is required on the first visit? ❑ full ❑ minimum of $_____ ❑ share of cost above insurance deductible ❑ other. Will you charge for consultation? ❑ yes ❑ no. Will you charge for the first two visits together on the first visit if you examine the first visit and treat the second? ❑ yes ❑ no How much? $_____

❑ 7. Will you charge for a Report of Findings? ❑ yes ❑ no ❑ how much? $_____

❑ 8. Will the patient pay you for outside consultation or specialists' fees? ❑ yes ❑ no or will the patient be responsible for covering these fees directly with the other practitioner (s)? ❑ yes ❑ no

❑ 9. What are the allowable forms of payment? ❑ cash ❑ check ❑ money order ❑ Visa ❑ Mastercard ❑ post dated checks ❑ payment plan ❑ bank loan ❑ parent payment

❑ 10. Is the patient responsible for the total amount of the fee? ❑ yes ❑ no. Do ❑ you or ❑ the patient bill a third party for payment? Will you absorb the difference if payment by third party is not in full? ❑ yes ❑ no. Will the patients pay the difference? ❑ yes ❑ no. How long will you extend credit before payment is re❑uired? ❑ no credit ❑ 30 ❑ 45 ❑ 60 ❑ 75 ❑ 90 days.

❑ 11. What is your office policy on insurance? Do you accept assignment of benefits? ❑ yes ❑ no. Is ❑ a full fee due now, or ❑ just an estimated deductible? Do ❑ you bill, or does ❑ the patient bill? If you bill, do you charge a service fee for filling out more than one form? ❑ yes ❑ no. If so, how much? $_____. If you participate in insurance programs or preferred provider programs, how are these programs handled differently? What is your policy on verifying insurance coverage? Will ❑ the patient verify and fill out a special form to submit to you, or will ❑ you verify coverage from within your office? If you verify insurance coverage, in what types of situations? ❑ Workers' Compensation? ❑ other? How will you communicate your insurance policy to patients? ❑ office brochure ❑ verbally by office staff ❑ patient letter. How will you verify their understanding and commitment to abide by your policy? ❑ verbally ❑ recorded on patient ledger or computer file ❑ signed policy and financial agreement statement.

❑ 12. Will you accept Medicare assignment? ❑ yes ❑ no (this is not even advisable until Medicare covers acupuncture.) or, will you have the patients pay you direct and have them bill Medicare? Will you accept state assistance program coverage? ❑ yes ❑ no. If so, how will you handle this? Will ❑ you bill or ❑ the patient bill?

13. If you initiate a payment plan with a patient, what is the maximum amount of payments allowed?_____ . Will you use ❑ promissory notes or truth in lending forms? Will you ❑ have them hand write an agree-ment? or ❑ will you have them sign your office payment plan agree ment. When will you allow a payment plan policy with a patient? Over $_____ of services rendered ❑ cases where the patient has proved consistency in paying ❑ other. What is the minimum payment pe month you will allow? $_____

14. Will you bill patients ❑ not at all ❑ monthly ❑ twice monthly? When would you not bill? ❑ outside collection service accounts ❑ zero balance ❑ other. What would be your billing cycle, if you do bill? ❑ 1st   and 3rd Wednesdays ❑ 7th and 21st of the month ❑ other.

15. Will you add ❑ interest or ❑ a service charge for rebilling? At what rate? ❑ fixed % rate ❑ flat rate. What rebilling charge will you assign? ❑ fixed % rate ❑ flat rate. After how many days? ❑ 30 ❑ 45 ❑ 60 ❑ 75 ❑ 90 days.

16. Will you accept litigation cases? ❑ yes ❑ no. Will you require the patient to cover any fees before the case is settled? ❑ yes ❑ no. What forms will you require them to sign? ❑ liens ❑ authorization to treat ❑ authorization to pay for reports ❑ other. When will you collect for fees in these cases? ❑ as services are rendered ❑ partial payment ❑ payment plan ❑ at settlement. Who pays the report fees? ❑ patient ❑ other. When? ❑ as services are rendered ❑ at settlement.

17. Will you charge for missed appointments? ❑ yes ❑ no ❑ sometimes ❑ after 24 hours notice? ❑ after the first missed appointment? ❑ after thesecond missed appointment ❑ if poor excuse? How will you notify patients if you do charge? ❑ office brochure ❑ sign at front desk ❑ on phone ❑ at the front desk when making next payment. How much will you charge? ❑ flat fee ❑ the cost if service was rendered.

18. Will you send accounts out for collections? ❑ yes ❑ no. When? ❑ 60 days ❑ 75 days ❑ 90 days ❑ other. Will you do collection calls within the office? ❑ collection letters? Will you ❑ use a collection service? How much will you still collect? _____%.

OPERATIONS

How to Set Up Your Bookkeeping System

A bookkeeping system can be simple or complex, according to what information you want to access. Basically, it involves:

Accounts Receivable: Accounting for monies owed, charged and paid.
Accounts Payable: Office Expenditures.
Patient Management: Control Statistics

You will need special summary computer printouts (or worksheets filled in manually) for tax purposes, as well as for practice management control. Your bookkeeper can record the data for you. These are the forms you will need:

1. Aging of accounts receivable sheets (Show where receivables are tied up) 1
2. Patient log of account number, numbers of patients 2
3. Appointment statistics, daily, weekly 1
4. Petty cash ledger 2
5. Payroll ledger
6. Equipment ledger and depreciation file or worksheet
7. Year End expenditure summary 1
8. Profit and loss statement 1
9. Monthly summary statistics 1

Most of these are included in the *Big Forms Packet* or in **Volume II** with specific instructions for using your accounts receivable and payable systems. Hire a good office manager who is well versed in accounting procedures to handle the daily details of keeping your records accurate and up to date. Simply get an overall sense of:

1. How manual and computer accounting systems work.
2. What is involved in using the accounts receivable and payable systems.
3. What forms you will need.

What bookkeeping system works best for you should be considered carefully before purchasing your financial system.

1 In the Big Forms Packet
2 In Volume II

Criteria for a Good Bookkeeping System

USE THE BELOW 10 BOOKKEEPING REQUIREMENTS AS A CHECKLIST.

No matter what system you use or group of forms you use, your bookkeeping system must::

■ 1. Fit with your financial policy. Your financial policy will determine how simple the accounts receivable system and insurance billing system will be.

■ 2. Most effectively increase your profitability, fit your budget, and be cost effective.

■ 3. Meet short range goals and needs as well as be considered in long range goal planning. Does it fit in volume of your practice now and your intention and plans for practice growth?

■ 4. Be the most time saving and effective for your purposes.

■ 5. Have a built in system to check accuracy.

■ 6. Provide immediate access to financial (and insurance) information for both patients' needs and yours.

■ 7. Be easy to use:

   ■ Is it unencumbered by lots of forms and paperwork?

   ■ Can it be used by more than one person simultaneously or in shifts?

   ■ Can you replace personnel easily using this system, i.e., if your staff went on vacation or quit?

■ 8. Be easy to understand:

   ■ How much time does it take to train into this system and be relatively error-free?_____

   ■ How committed is your staff to using this system?
   _____

■ 9. Have a back up plan for using the system:

   ■ 1. Train more than one front office staff member how to use it.

   ■ 2. Know the system yourself.

   ■ 3. Have duplicate day sheets in a safe place or a back up disc for the computer, both of which can be used in case originals are damaged.

■ 10. Be as much as possible, an all data base system where information can be plugged simultaneously into many of the computer file or forms listed previously.

   ■ How many steps can be saved by one system over another?

   ■ With the system you use, how much time does it take to compute totals, correct errors, and transfer totals to different files or worksheets? How much time could be saved using this system over another?

   ■ Does it meet all your needs now? Will it later? Is it cost effective?

What to Choose — A Manual or Computer System?

There are two main systems that simultaneously record information, cut data processing time and the number of papers handled, as well as cut long range costs. They are the computer and the one-write pegboard system. In addition, you need to consider the most efficient insurance processing or billing system that goes with this. There are also combinations of the two systems which can be put together very effectively to meet your needs. This can get complex, so buying a system is best handled working with any combination of the following: practice management consultant, medical office manager skilled in such things, and a computer expert. Use the information in this chapter as a base for knowledge, as well as determining what kind of issues to address in purchasing your system.

Computers have many features in common. However, 1) some are better designed than others. 2) Some are all data based and have an automatic back up disc system to use in case the computer malfunctions or the material on the disc you are currently working with is destroyed or erased. 3) Some provide more of the functions you need and have already written medical software packages that would work for you. Check the software packages carefully. The software must do what you need. Get professional consultation on this. Don't buy a computer system unless the computer, software, megabyte size, and printer are right for your purposes and practice volume.

If you need an accounts receivable package and an accounts payable package:

❑ 1. Is there a checking system on the software packages so that you can be alerted and find errors in the event that the accounting system does not balance?

❑ 2. Is the system set up to record who paid and the date payments are received, in addition to the amount paid?

❑ 3. Is there a specialty insurance billing package included with the accounting package? (If there is, make sure the ICDA, CPT, and RVS billing codes are current, usable, complete, and appropriate for your state and situation.)

❑ 4. Can the computer you need print out individual bills and insurance forms, as well as batch hitting bills (If this serves your purpose)?

❑ 5. Can the system printout what the patient's share of cost is? Is there a way the computer bills this?

❑ 6. Does the all data base system you have easily or simultaneously plug the information you need into your practice management statistic files?

When you go to buy a computer, explore the additional programs or packages available for that computer now rather than later. Ask yourself:

❑ 1. "Do I want word processing capability to write my own letters and reports? Or do I need a setup word processing package for letter and report writing? Does what I have now serve my needs best?"

❏ 2. "If a patient letter series is included in a package that I want, does the tone and content of the letters represent me?"

❏ 3. "Do I want a program to create my own advertising and newsletter?"

If you do, you will need something like "Pagemaker," which is a desk top publishing program, which works on many compatible IBM and MacIntosh computers. You or your public relations person will need to be trained in how to use it. If your assistant is already trained, bravo! Ask at your local computer store about this program.

These and many other considerations can be looked at by you and an expert before you purchase your computer, printer, program or series of software packages. Notice that the all data base systems can do instant simultaneous functions which can record the same information at once into many different files of a software package. Information may simultaneously be input to go into the individual patient file, to the daily accounts receivable sheet, to batch hit billing, to aging analysis by patient and type of claim, to birthday print outs, to a recall file, to letter series, to weekly printouts, monthly summaries, and yearly summaries and distribution— invaluable practice statistics up to the minute. For the accounts payable, computers easily access totals in various expense areas of your practice so you can look at expense control.

Computers may involve less transposition of numbers by humans, may involve less time and cost of labor, as well as provide a multilevel type of function simultaneously that a pegboard system alone could not accomplish. One thing to remember: a system is only as useful to you and as accurate for you as it is programmed to be. Although there are excellent accuracy checks in the computer system, it is important that the ones who punch in information be accurate. Computers do not solve posting problems. You can run control adding machine tapes on all number totals. Make sure that the work inputted is double checked.

All pegboard systems have some features in common. The basic item of all pegboards is a pegboard, which is a fold out board with small metal pegs along the left side. A series of forms are punched to fit on these pegs, and these forms lay on the open board. The pegs allow all the forms to align for the speed of one writing. Some systems require carbon paper to duplicate entries. Others use coated carbonless paper which eliminate a messy situation. The "day sheets" which peg over onto these boards have proofing boxes to double check accuracy, can be set up to record daily, month to date, and year to date totals, as well as record distribution of service by type and by who rendered the service. The day sheets differ in design. These sheets require humans to compute, total, find errors, correct them, and transfer information to various practice management control sheets.

Both the computer systems (particularly the all database plug-ins) and the one-write pegboard systems:

1. Avoid rewriting the same information many times on separate forms;
2. Completely itemize each patient visit (accounts receivable) and expense (accounts payable).

Both systems are:

1. Easy to prove or balance;
2. Reduce errors; and
3. Assist in clarifying money messages and communications in the office when used with the proper forms.

In buying a pegboard system, note that the form companies which sell them vary in the cost of their systems, their ability to do custom work, as well as the level of service they offer. It is important to have a service representative from the company of your choice do the "follow-up" work so that you use whatever system you use correctly.

You will also want to consider adjuncts such as insurance billing and other options for your specific needs, so be sure you review the upcoming section for different options first before making purchasing decisions.

If you are starting in practice you will usually start with a manual system because the outlay of cash is far less. However, once you have advanced to a rapid growth stage, automate your system--particularly in practices with more than one practitioner.

The Accounts Payable System

The purpose of an accounts payable system is to provide an accurate accounting when 1) you are billed; 2) have an expense related to the business; 3) a payment is made; and 4) a balance is involved. Your accounts payable ledger is your record of deposits in and expenses out, your data for practice management control and income tax computing, as well as proof of your business activity.

It is recommended that you separate your business from your personal checking account to clarify what your business expenses are. After you choose your bank and open your business account, stop—before you order checks. You will need to order checks from a forms company if you use the one-write pegboard system because the pegboard checks fit over the pegs. Have your business name and your name and title printed on your checks, as well as your address, phone number, and social security number.

The "Cash Disbursement and Payroll Journal" with duplicate checks shingled and numbered, is an excellent one-write accounts payable pegboard system. The payroll sheets are useful for employee record keeping. There are many types on the market that vary in cost, labor and simplicity. Some involve less transposition of numbers. Some have proofing boxes for double checking your totals. Some do not.

Pegboard systems complete the posting simply by writing the check. Rather than having a separate check stub and record of distribution where entries are made at separate times, you end up with an actual carbon of the check and automatic recording onto your distribution page. You can take checks out without taking your pegboard with you. Just make sure you have recorded the basics and fill in the amount when you return. This system is designed to have the least amount of transposition errors and it is always up to date.

If you use a computer, all you need is your check register and your monthly statement with checks to punch information into the computer for accounts payable. I prefer duplicate checks. You may want to use the pegboard system with the computer as a backup system or the reverse. As long as you have a safely housed backup disc kept current, you are protected from loss of information if your original computer disc is destroyed and erased.

Purchasing, Inventory, and Ordering Set Up

Under the "Financial Planning" section, you had an opportunity to project your opening expenses and make an inventory list of what was needed, the amount, and the cost involved. The items which you purchase should be kept track of, not only on your general expense ledger, but on a separate ledger. Use an equipment ledger and depreciation worksheets. There may be large enough purchases and long-life purchases which would not be a direct expense write off, but be written off over a period of years. See a tax consultant regarding how to depreciate for tax purposes; or, have your bookkeeping person fill you in on these details if he or she is knowledgeable in this area. You can also consult the local IRS office itself if you have any questions. Their advice is free.

In the U.S. you will not normally need a retail sales license if you have already paid tax on the item to the company and are including the product as part of your treatment rendered. However, you probably will be required to obtain a U.S. retail sales licence if you do sales, do not pay tax to the supplier, and pass the tax to the consumer. Check with your supplier on this and your local and state tax office to see what is appropriate in your case. Also, check with your supplier on what is the usual, customary, and reasonable mark up on supplies the supplier sells you. It often ranges from 50-100%.

Keep a rolodex or list of from whom you buy equipment and supplies, as well as your account number with your suppliers. If you don't have one, establish credit with them. Set up your "Suppliers List" as follows:

Name of Supp.	Address	Phone	Acct.#	Type of Supp.	Discount offered	Delivery Time	Freight Charge	Fill-in Policy

Who pays? You, the buyer? Your leasing company? On which items? On what terms?

Note: Purchasing herbs and acupuncture devices from abroad is under special regulation of the Food and Drug Administration. Get a copy of the regulations for purchase and resale. Address: Food and Drug Administration, Washington, D. C.

Inventory Management

1. It is important to keep all orders updated so emphasize this to your staff, particularly those herbs, teas, etc. which you use as part of your treatment. It is important to have enough inventory on hand for hoe care and patient sales. Keep an eye out on the stock levels and keep a record of your inventory. For any item there is a maximum stock level, a minimum stock level and a reorder point. There are computer programs designed to track this. Have your assistant be aware of these levels for ordering purposes

2. A combination "Retail Price List and Ordering Sheet" can be used: 1) as a front desk price list for patients, 2) to keep track of your inventory and what needs to be ordered, and 3) to assess what you have on order and for what you are waiting. One way of keeping track of your cost and retail inventory is to make a notebook with dividers marked A-Z with a list of your supplies by the first letter of the supply item in English and Chinese, for example, etc., as below:

Item Eng./Chin.	Ordered from	Our Cost	Patient's Cost
XX100	XXX	$3.00	$6.00

3. Emphasize to your staff when ordering by phone to communicate both the English and Chinese (or other name) of herbs ordered to avoid misunderstandings with the herb companies. The name of the person spoken to at the herb company should be recorded, as well as what was ordered, the date, English and oriental name, amount, cost, and the expected delivery date. When you receive supplies, check the packing slip against the order. Keep the packing slips, which will be matched to the invoices for payment.

4. Whoever fills formulas should be given <u>specific</u> instructions in proper preparation and care and should be cautioned on any malpractice implications. All products should be carefully labeled with the patient's name, what's in the bottle, and <u>written</u> instructions for use.

5. Do not overstock. Preparations can go bad! It also ties up your financial resources. Every dollar of excess inventory is every dollar not available for use. Keep track. Runaway inventories can be a threat to liquid assets.

6. Markup adds cash and cash flow to your practice. Keep a record of your prices to the patient, as well as the amount of monthly sales generated. Note the inventory list on page 140. Expand the amount and types of items with your practice needs and as your financial base improves.

The Accounts Receivable System

The purpose of an accounts receivable system is to provide an accurate accounting when a patient is charged for services rendered, a payment is made, and a balance is involved. You use ledger cards, fee slips and superbills, as well as a "Control, Aging, and Analysis Sheet" with this system. These records are vital for the following reasons:

* They provide a means for clear business dealings.
* They are your proof of receipt of payment and adjustments.
* They record the amount of cash flow into your practice.
* They are a tool for use in maintaining practice management control.
* They provide proof of accuracy for audit and income tax purposes.

There are THREE MAJOR ACCOUNTS RECEIVABLE SYSTEMS:

■ 1. An in-office computer (all data base preferred) with 1-2 terminals.

■ 2. Out-of-Office computerized billing/management control system. (Some systems are attached to the duplicate day sheet pegboard system. Some systems are set-up to use with ledgers in-office with an appropriate fee slip.)

■ 3. In-office one-write pegboard system with peg over insurance billing forms.

In addition to daily accounts receivable pegboard sheets, you will need to include:

1. Ledger cards with a ledger tray.
Use multipurpose and either one or both sided ledgers. Also NCR coated ledgers are preferred for pegboard systems.

■ They are used in order to balance against open balances on computers or day sheets, as well as double check the daily payments and fees.

- They can provide a monthly statement or a photocopied receipt to patient.
- They provide immediate access to the patient's financial status.

- They provide an itemized up to date accounting of services, charges, payments made, balance.

- They are invaluable for: recording insurance information (on the top part of ledger), fast recording on superbills, recording when superbills are given to the patient or are sent to insurance companies, and when payment is due next.

- They are a record of the financial arrangement.

2. Bank deposit slips.
(NCR coated deposit slips can slip over the daysheets.)

- They should be in duplicate, one for the bank and one for the office.

- Deposit slips with the pegboard system. One-write recording is done at the time of service. The top deposit slip is attached to your regular bank deposit slip with "total only" recorded on your regular slip.

3. Computer Billing Statements.
These can be used in lieu of ledger cards for billing.

- You will feed the data regarding your patient into your computer. You can either a) give the the billing to the patient at the time of service or b) "batch hit" on the computer when you want to generate a number of bills and send them to the patients or insurance companies. If you use an out-of-office computer company, follow their instructions.

4. Fee Slips.
- These are the intercommunication money and message slips between the acupuncturist and the front office staff, which should be used with either computer or pegboard systems. They can be designed and used as a single fee slip or used as a combination superbill and fee slip, whichever fits (See **Volume II** for sample).

5. Insurance "Practitioner's Statement" and Billing Forms.
- These must usually be custom printed with the current RVS/CPT

service codes and ICDA diagnostic codes that are most appropriate for your use. (The masters are in the Insurance Forms Packet. From Tao to Earth, Focus PM Distribution. also does custsomized work on masters.)

■ Superbills are specifically designed for efficient billing done by the patient (or by the office) and are adapted to be included or attached to the individual's patient claim form. Some "peg over" and receipt.

■ It is important to be aware of which companies require special billing forms such as Blue Cross/Blue Shield and state or federal aid. (These do not have a receipt).

■ Be aware that there is a "Universal Claim Form" which can be made to be "more efficient" than typed in full each time. These do not "peg over" or receipt. It is not the most efficiently expedient form to use unless they are used in batch hit computer printouts.

6. Appointment Cards
■ These can be adapted onto other forms such as patient receipt or superbill combinations.

■ When given separately, they can be best adapted for multiple appointments. They provide great advertising with your name and a statement like "We Care". They can also be combined with a fold over "Courtesy consultation for a friend or family member at our office".

Each of these forms require decisions on your part as to what you want on these forms. I have provided some examples. However, because of the myriad of choices within the six categories above, it is invaluable to have feedback and assistance from a forms company representative, someone who is trained in medical software accounts receivable programs, and/or a practice management consultant to assist you in person with the purchase and training in setting up your system. This is true even if your office assistant has used an accounts receivable system before. You will want to make sure that the system you choose is being implemented properly. Some forms company representatives will offer you the service of checking in with you to see if you need more forms and to answer any questions regarding the use of the system. The representatives and some of the medical software companies, are also available to answer your questions by phone. Use this service as you need it. Most companies include this at no charge as part of their service.

Choosing Your Billing Systems

Below are several kinds of billing systems, among which one or a combination will work best for your practice.

Ledger Billing*
Ledger billing is the most common form of billing in the office. A photocopy of the patients financial ledger card is sent to cash paying and insurance patients alike on a monthly basis. Insurance patients are checked mid month to inform those patients who have 45 day accounts and to let them know if their insurance company has paid. You only need access to a photocopy machine to do ledger billing.

Universal Claim Form System
Universal claim forms are mostly used in offices that do all insurance claims. They are not a substitute for the insurance company's claim form. They are used like a superbill and are not as efficient as a superbill unless printed out by a computer. Then they are extremely efficient. Computer claim forms are used by practices in the growth phase of practice expansion.

Superbills
Superbills are as widely used as are the Universal Claim Forms. Practice management and insurance management seminars either advocate or admonish them. Take a look at the advantages or disadvantages and the appropriateness of using them in your particular practice.

Superbills can be designed:
1. To be quickly processed at the time of service.

2. To be professional.
   Neat when hand written on.
   Simplify and accurately reflect::
   ■ Correct coding
   ■ Services, dates, charges
   ■ Patient information
   ■ Diagnosis

* In the *Big Forms Packet*

3. To be visually easy to read and process by insurance companies.

4. To be easy to attach by the patient to her/his insurance claim form.

5. To not require the office to process the claim form:
   - Cuts the amount of paperwork
   - Cuts information checking
   - Cuts filing time
   - Cuts typing time
   - Cuts photocopying time
   - Cuts the cost of personal time
   - Cuts the cost of paper printing and envelopes
   - Cuts the cost of photocopying, photocopy paper, and stamps

6. To be an instant bill. No waiting involved to submit it.

7. To be efficient, particularly the ones with five spaces for services.

8. To reflect clear financial agreement (with signed assignment of benefits).

9. To be easily bookkept and checked on when using interfacing systems. It also can be easily redone if there are errors on it.

10. To interface with pegboard system, ledger cards, and/or with a computer system.

Contrary to some insurance management firms, I have found that insurance companies do not generally discriminate against superbill use -- particularly when it is attached to the patient's claim form. Blue Cross and Blue Shield, however, prefer their own forms typed in. They look like the Universal Claim Form. Their reasoning is that superbills have not generally been uniform; their processors have to hunt for all the information, and the formats of many superbills don't contain all the essential information to process the claim, so the claims are delayed and returned for more information. A well designed superbill, such as the one in the *Big Forms Packet*, solves the problem. They are excellent for new practices or growth phase practices.

In-Office Computerized Billing
If you can afford a computer, this is usually your most effective and efficient system for high patient volume practices where billing is done monthly by the

office and not the patients. Offices in a growth or expansion phase will usually move into in-office computerized billing.

Out-Of-Office Computerized Billing

I have noticed a number of offices where a great deal of in-office time is involved in double checking and correcting these billings -- mostly because staff inputted or forgot to input the correct information. Also, there are two main problems:

1. There is delay in the computer company redoing billings or

2. There is a delay with in-office hand typing of missed information needed on these forms.

However, if you are a new practitioner, without staff, and use a basic fee slip such as the one in **Volume II**, out of office billing may be your most efficient, time saving, and cost effective route for billing. Check in your local area for a medical billing service.

Whatever system you use, the key to billing management is to stay on top of billing. Staying on top of billing keeps cash flow moving--critical for all practices and even more so at the beginning stages. Bill patients at least once a month with ledger bills and/or at the same time of service with superbills. Don't let insurance billing get behind longer than three days or over $300 per billing.

Consideration on Who Bills Insurance

Patients either pay by cash, Visa, Mastercard, and or have their bills paid substantially through various health plans—either private or public insurance programs such as Medicare, Blue Cross, Blue Shield, Workers' Compensation and Personal Injury Coverage. Billing the insurance companies can occur in a variety of ways. Basically the three most utilized approaches are:

1. The office does all the insurance billings.
2. The patient does the insurance billing.
3. The office takes care of 100% coverage billing such as Workers' Compensation, Personal Injury and Litigation and allows the patient to bill general insurance.

The rationale most often taken for the office doing all billing is:
1. It is a courtesy to the patient.

2. The office wants to have control over processing the claim forms so that the billing is completed and benefits are clearly assigned to the office.

The rationale for patient doing the insurance billing is:
1. The overhead cost of incorporating a part or full time insurance department is prohibitive or costly. Dollars may be more profitably used in other areas of the practice.

2. If the patients bill, the staff can be freer to attend to more personal patient care and spend less time on the "paper chase"—trying to keep up with the paperwork.

3. Patients can easily attach a superbill to their claim form. (A superbill is simply a doctor's statement or practitioner's statement that gives the insurance companies the necessary information in most cases to reimburse charges and payments).

4. Patients are pleased because they can send their bills in far more quickly than the office insurance department can get them out.

5. Patients have control over when the insurance claims go in and the claims being done properly. The office has control over the agreement established as to when full payment is due (See Financial Policies section) and when partial payment is due by the patient. The office can still implement insurance handling effectively without having to spend a large amount of time processing individually.

The rationale behind the office taking care of part of the insurance: (Workers' compensation, personal injury cases and 100% coverage by insurance companies, such as in the case of accidents.)

1. Many of these cases require extra reporting in addition to the doctor's or practitioner's statement. These reports must accompany forms which the individual insurance company uses. These reports need to be on file and may require follow-up work.

2. The office wants to have control over 100% payment from the insurance company direct to the practitioner.

I know of highly successful practitioners who have an all cash practice who allow their patients to do their own billing. I also know of highly successful practitioners who are equally as successful and who do all of the billing. Their patient has only to meet his/her deductibles and percentages not covered by the insurance policy. There are practices who blend a combination of accepting assignment and allowing the patient to take responsibility for their bill and also are highly successful. What makes a difference in the success of the practice is:

■ The attitude of service behind these office policies and the consistency by the staff in being of service.

■ The reduction of stress because of using the particular policy.

■ The fact that a particular policy promotes patient follow-through care and still meets the cash flow needs of the practice.

If doing all the billing within the office creates stress and takes away from patient care, it doesn't fit. If handling cases involving reports best serves to bill within the office, do so. Asking Medicare patients to do their own billing fits right now, because acupuncture is not covered by Medicare at this time. Usually Medicare billing done within the office can greatly assist older patients who have a difficult time writing or seeing. If you notice a patient is disabled and has no one to assist him/her with billing, please assist him/her out of courtesy. Because insurance can be so complex to keep on track, patients willing to accept responsibility for their personal agreements with their insurance companies are greatly encouraged through office policy to do so.

In the beginning of practice make sure you have a solid cash flow. You will out of necessity ask for cash or credit card payments up front and give your patients a superbill. "As your practice flow is stabilized, liberalize and consider only requiring 50% payment at the time of service for those who assign insurance benefits to you. In the expansive phase of your practice, loosen your policy fully to patient payment of the percentage of copayment (after the patients's deductible on his policy is met.)

If you take the time to set up your insurance system ahead of time, you will open up greater possibilities for your patients to complete their care. A good liberalized, well-organized insurance system can serve to increase your practice growth about 80%, according to Dr. Peter G. Fernandez's studies of practitioners who expected those returns.

Accounting and Billing Summary

Either computer or manual systems require decisions on your part as to what equipment, billing systems, and forms you want to use, and how much you can afford to outlay in consideration of upcoming cash flow needs. The information provided in this section gives you the information to make accounting set up decisions, billing decisions, and be a more educated buyer. Now you are ready to get feedback and assistance from someone who is trained in medical software accounts receivable programs, and a forms company representative to assist you in person with the purchase and training in setting up your system. It is still advisable to have outside input and assistance even if your office assistant has used an accounts receivable system before.

You will want to make sure that the system you choose is being implemented properly. Office forms companies such as Safeguard, Bibbero, and Practice Efficiency in California are among many companies which provide ongoing service to their customers.

An outside local billing company, can further present the case for out of office billing, especially for new practitioners without staff, and help you with your questions as well.

When you contact your local office forms company to help you in setting up your billing systems and forms, you can show their representative the masters from the forms packets, which either they can print or a printer can print for you. From Tao to Earth Focus Practice Management does do custom work for those who purchase their forms packets. From Tao to Earth's rates are substantially cheaper than forms company setups for their masters. Take advantage of the fact that forms company representatives can also answer questions that have been stimulated by reading about these systems and forms in the packets, and they are happy to assist.

Note: Procedures for implementing the daily accounting and billing systems are detailed in **Volume II.**

Your Accounting and Billing System

Will you use a manual system, or a computer system? _____
_____

What billing system will you use? _____
_____
_____

Who will do the billing? _____

What parts of the system will you need to purchase and what is the cost?

_____   _____
_____   _____
_____   _____
_____   _____
_____   _____
_____   _____
_____   _____
_____   _____
_____   _____
_____   _____

What is the total cost of your accounting system? _____
_____

What is the cost of your billing system? _____
_____

How will you finance it? _____
_____

Will your initial accounting purchase or lease costs save time, energy and
money overall in labor efficiency or in services you can provide? Yes ❑
No ❑ Is your billing system the best for you now? Yes ❑ No ❑ Will you
review it for change in the next year? Yes ❑ No ❑   _____
_____

Patient and Practice Management Forms Use

Purchasing Your Forms

When you set up your practice, purchase the forms you need before you open if possible. Many practices try to create their forms as they go, which is both time consuming, exhausting, and may not save you in the long run. Whether you are a starting practitioner or established, From Tao to Earth Focus Practice Management now has available forms designed and carefully thought through, specifically for acupuncturists. [1]

Setting Your Procedure and Policy for Form Use

Thoroughly understanding the "18 Ways to Increase Safe Practice Communications ," "Safe Practice Guidelines and Policies (Reducing Malpractice Vulnerability" and "The Value of Continuing Care Scheduling" will show you how your forms can be used to enhance and reinforce maximum good patient care.

Forms Use As An Asset for Practice Growth

The way specific forms can be used can determine and increase practitioner acceptance and safe practice, avoid misunderstandings, reinforce patient follow-through, and set new patterning of health for patients.[2] They also add to practice growth. Dr. Peter G. Fernandez has carefully studied health care providers and discovered some percentages in expected practice increase from using good patient care procedures with the forms use.

40%	Written Report --Recommendations and Instructions
up to	With Recommended schedule (intensified care **25%**, corrective
195%	care **100%**, rehabilitation **40%**, maintenance care **30%**)

30%	Multiple Appointment Card Use
10%	Patient Reminder Cards Use (with calls)

Dr. Fernandez Found these percentages additionally:

10%	**Patient Letters** sent out regularly, including thank you for refer-ring letter, introduction to your office and care, referral material
80%	**Insurance forms** with a liberalized insurance program

Up to a **365%** increase in practice growth!

[1] The "Big Forms Packet" $48.00 (or $39.75 for those who purchase Volume I) is for "mixing and matching" forms you use in your practice.

The "Insurance Forms Packet" $28.50 is the complement for handling the insurance part of your practice. (Further explanation for insurance use is in Volume II and Volume III of the series.)

The appointment management forms provide safe practice, ease in patient flow and appointment control necessary to assess 1) Patient volume and 2) increase and decrease in volume.

The financial management control forms are immeasurable in value as they provide the statistics to guide your practice and manage adjustments.

Staff hiring forms and contracts are essential for clear agreements, vital to protect your investment of time, energy, and money.

The Big Forms Table of Contents

CONTINUED NEXT PAGE   PM69 c. C. Flint Bestani

Big Forms Packet
From Tao to Earth Focus Practice
Management Publications Distribution
To order: Call 1 (800) 800-3139
Mastercard/Visa accepted.

```
┌─────────────────────────┐
│                         │
│    The Acupuncturist's  │
│                         │
│       Insurance         │
│     Forms Packet        │
│                         │
│                         │
│                         │
│                         │
│   by Cynthia Flint Bestani │
│                         │
└─────────────────────────┘
```

The Insurance Forms Packet Includes:

Insurance Forms Roster & Basic Instructions

Patient Preparation for Insurance Billing
PM140   Welcome Brochure & Office Policy
PM26/   Patient Registration (2pp)
PM27
PM23B   New Patient Information on Insurance
PM18   Insurance Questions and Answers for
          Patients
PM23A   How to Submit Your Insurance Claim
PM48/49   Verification of Insurance Coverage for
          Acupuncture — 2 pages

Re: Obtaining Coverage
PM20   Re: Coverage of Acupuncture by

          Licensed Acupuncturists in CA.
PM61-I   Coverage of Acupuncture Letter to

          Individuals and companies
PM19   Petition for Acupuncture Coverage

Authorizations for General Insurance Coverage
PM35A   Authorization to Release Medical

          Information
PM35B   Physician Referral for Acupuncture
PM23b   Preauthorization for Treatment by
          Insurance Carrier

Insurance Billing and Accounting Forms
PML113   One visit Superbill
PM119   5 Visit Superbill
UNIV   Universal Claim Form
PML1   Insurance Control Form for Recording
          billing, payments, & tracking
PM172   Sample Ledger Card

Financial Agreement Re: Insurance Payment
PM14   Notice of Liability to Insurance Co.
          and Patient's Attorney
PM14   Irrevocable Assignment of Benefits
PM8   Power of Attorney to Endorse Checks
          to the Office/ Practitioner
PM21   60 Days Extension of Credit in Consid-
          eration of Assignment
PM17   Deductible Coverage Policy for Patients
PM16   60 Days 'Payment Letter to Patient

Further Insurance Tracking
PM7   Duplicate Superbill. Advise status.
PM15   Insurance Tracer
PM6   Take Action Letter

**Auto, Personal Injury, Work Injury
History/Agreements**
PM174/5   Accidental Injury Questionnaire
PM62   Automobile/Work Injury Policy
          Statement
PM12   Personal Injury Financial Policy
PM13   Re: Medical Reports and Acupuncturist's
          Lien
PM51   Statement of Report Charges (and
          agreement of coverage by patient
          insurance companies, and/or attorney)

Reports for Insurance
P183   Patient Fill-In Progress Report
          (Patient Evidence)
PM46   Treatment Summary Report
P186   Initial Report
P187   Interim and Final Report
PM300   Complete Narrative Report 5 pages

Workers' Compensation
PM75   Workers' Compensation Worksheet
PM173   Workers' Compensation Questionnaire
PM34   Letter of Authorization to Employer for
          Workers' Compensation
Copy   Notice and Request for Allowance of
          Lien Workers' Compensation
Copy   Doctor's First Report of Injury -
          Workers' Compensation
Copy   Monthly (and Final) Billing Form
Copy   Application for Adjudication of Claim
Copy   Declaration of Readiness to Proceed

PM71A revised edition,copyright 199? C.Flint Bestani
Insurance Forms Packet : $28.50 Plus $8.00 U.S. Shipping
From Tao to Earth Focus Practice Mgmt. Pubs Distribution
To ORDER Call: 1 (800) 800-3139

Purchasing Scheduling Aids

The "Appointment Book Log Book" can be ordered through many of the forms company representatives, or you can buy one through a stationary story. If you like the appointment log sheet in the *Big Forms Packet* and it fits your time increments for scheduling, the page can be photocopied on white or various colored pages and whole punched and put into a notebook.

The forms company appointment logs often come color coded (a different color for each day) and shingled so that you can flip through the days of the week more easily. This is advantageous if you have a very busy practice and where appointments are scheduled for one or more practitioners. Order the appointment book so you get the appointment spacing you need. For example, appointment books are set up so that the increments for scheduling are in either ten minute, fifteen minute, or twenty minute intervals. What kind of time intervals would fit your type of practice?

Creative visualization of the appointment book is an important aspect of scheduling, as you will see in the upcoming sections, so take the time to buy the best. Whoever schedules your appointments is likely to spend a great deal of his/ her time on the phone or at the desk scheduling. We know that color affects attitude, so the rainbow colored pages-appointment book would enhance positive and creative energy flow. This may seem like a small point now, but later you will be able to appreciate the effect. Little pleasures like these can also provide the positive and bright reminders that shift your focus in times when you most need it.

Scheduling aids which will assist you in carrying out the procedures such as discussed in this upcoming section, are available in the *Big Forms Packet*:

Personal Acupuncture Report, Schedule, & Recommendations
Appointment Log Sheet
Sign-In Register Sheet
Multiple Appointment Cards with Reevaluation Time
Reminder Cards
Appointment cards for Courtesy Consultation
Appointment Card for courtesy treatment for Referring a Patient
Appt. Card for Our Orientation &Acupuncture Health Care Class
Appointment Card for Referral Out for (lab work, consultation, other)

INSURANCE, REPORTING, AND COURT PREPARATION

Dealing With the Insurance Situation

Insurance payment for acupuncture is not available that we know of, in states which do not license acupuncturists. The movement toward insurance coverage, then is preceded by licensing acupuncturists first in that state.

Because acupuncture is still so little understood in this country, including the outstanding results with treatment, it will take educating the public, the legal system, medical doctors, and researches of its benefits and safety. It is still considered an "experimental procedure" in the U.S. by the FDA.

Business executives are putting the high cost of health care under the microscope these days and they don't like what they see. Health care now consumes 10.5% of the gross national product. Twenty five years ago, it was 5% in the U.S. Ten years from now, it is estimated to be 15% – if the present rate of increase continues. If acupuncture can show how to significantly decrease health care costs per capita, acupuncture will be more apt to be supported by insurance companies, as well as be included in the new way of the future, good or bad – Preferred Provider Organizations. It is up to acupuncturists to stand together through their national and state organizations so that those who make major decisions which affect every acupuncturist's practice, can be influenced by the collective funds and endeavor of the acupuncturist profession.

We have found that practices increase 80% by the use of insurance billing procedures. Hence, in order to get more patients under care, and under care which can allow a consistency of treatment, insurance seems to be one of the best resources to serve people. It also provides the stability of most practices economically. You can see how important it is to participate in your state and national associations who are active politically in getting laws passed which will favor insurance coverage of acupuncture.

Even in those states which have been more victorious in acupuncture coverage, insurance companies seem to lag somewhat behind legal changes. It can take both patience and persistence in obtaining payment from individual companies. Most states still will only permit insurance coverage by physician referral of an M.D., D.C. or D.O. Workers' compensation companies who use RVS coding which includes acupuncture, tend to pay more consistently than the individual or group policies. Many companies in states which authorize payment to acupuncturists by insurance companies need to be reminded of current law from time to time. You may find your front office staff needs to use such aids as the preprinted letters with your billings. (There is a letter included in the *Insurance Forms Packet* for this purpose to remind the insurance company of their responsibility for coverage.)

To save yourself wasted time, energy, and money, have your patients call their insurance company and fill in the "Verification of Insurance Coverage Form" first to determine if acupuncture is covered on their policy. If it is not, there are some alternatives for the future. Presently in the *Insurance Forms Packet* there is a petition and letter to employers requesting acupuncture coverage for their individual employees. Your front office insurance biller can give these to patients to submit to their companies.

If you are sure in your state that dealing with insurance companies is not worth it to you, have your patients agree to pay you at the time services are rendered, either by cash, check, or Mastercard/Visa, and have the insurance company reimburse them. Mastercard/Visa gives them some grace before the insurance company reimburses them. Because general insurance contracts are a contract between the patient and the insurance company, and not between the practitioner and the insurance company, any disputes are rightly handled between the patient and the insurance company. You can assist by clarifying any points of unclarity.

If letters to the individual insurance company don't help your patients regarding reimbursement for health care services, your patients may choose small claims court or a report to the insurance commission in the state which mandates acupuncture coverage by insurance companies.

Insurance companies in the U.S. know about disease and illness. They do not pay for preventative care, in most cases. The protocol and the law states that you must have as assessment, diagnosis, prognosis and a treatment plan. The insurance company needs treatment procedure.

Procedure: Course of action or process going on in reference to a mode or method. A procedure tells the insurance company what the acupuncturist does.

Diagnosis: To distinguish the nature of the condition through examination.

An important area is accepted nomenclature. This is defined as whatever the specific insurance company accepts. There are a few important publications to use when deciding on diagnostic and procedure code nomenclature. Refer to the section of Volume I and II on "How to Procedure Code Your Services." You will need to purchase an ICD-9-CM set.

In **Volume III Success with Insurance** your assistant will learn how to handle patient insurance intake procedure, billing and follow-up procedures. Step by step instructions are included in Volume II for how to fill out the forms.

It is helpful for you to know the following: Many practitioners give their patients an option if they have insurance. That option is either to pay at the time of service and be reimbursed by their insurance company, or to sign what is called "Assignment of Benefits." This is a statement which in essence says that the patient authorizes the insurance company to pay you directly for services rendered. If you use the "Assignment of Benefits" approach, it is vital to use it with an insurance assignment policy which you set up in your office. The patient can read and have explained by your staff exactly how your financial policy works. It is not a good business practice to wait indefinitely for payment. You would have big cash flow problems in that event. It is often recommended that you extend assignment of insurance with a 60 day grace period, with partial payment by the patient each visit (consider the stage of practice you are at before setting the percentage of patient payment required at the time of services). Partial payment generally covers that part of your bill which insurance will not cover. Office financial policies for insurance vary from full payment by the patient each visit to 50% to 20% of covered services per visit. Patient policies will not normally cover herbs, vitamins, or supplements, so these must be covered at the time of services. Further explanation is included in **Volume II** for the benefit of your assistant. All the insurance forms for carrying out insurance are included in the *Insurance Forms Packet.*

As a practitioner, insurance billing is one area that is a daily routine procedure which you must let go and delegate. It is simply too time-consuming for you to handle insurance and all its ins and outs. With the exception of reporting, all other insurance procedures can and should be handled by a front office assistant or a part/full time insurance clerk who has had some background already in handling insurance. If you have never done insurance before, it's not a good idea to hire someone who knows less than you do about it. Start by hiring a part time insurance clerk-someone who does billing in another medical office. Perhaps someone who wants to moonlight. There are many areas of practice management that you can give your attention to which produce greater results for your time and much less aggravation.

What you can do is to make sure those areas which cause issue with insurance companies are handled. I have listed those in outline form so you can see what they are and how they can be solved. Where insurance covers acupuncture, the solutions provided will optimize insurance reimbursement.

Optimze Insurance Payment

MINIMIZE THE FOLLOWING DISPUTABLE INSURANCE COMPANY ISSUES

ISSUE	SUGGESTED SOLUTION
Gaps in Patient History	1. Be sure the patient fills in a complete history form, work injury, personal or auto injury questionnaires, if it applies. Insurance companies in review are trained to notice discrepancies in patient histories, correlating treatments, and results. They look to see if what the patient has said previously about his health matches current statements and if what you indicate matches what patients say about their health.
Proper Diagnosis	2. The patient should be given a proper and full diagnosis. Avoid shortchanging the patient in such ways as shortening the diagnosis or being unspecific diagnostically on the patient's claim form or practitioner's statement.
Unclear Diagnosis	3. If needed, use a stated "tentative diagnosis or working diagnosis" until confirming your diagnosis. This lets the insurance company know the diagnosis may change. Tentative diagnosis are often done when awaiting laboratory findings.
Diagnosis not commensurate with injury or illness.	4. Use diagnostic corollaries in reporting. A diagnostic corollary states the patient's complaint, the examination finding, the ICD-9-CM modifying diagnosis with numerical code, and major diagnosis radiographic and/or thermographic findings. A copy of fully completed examination forms can back you up if correct diagnosis becomes an issue. If you don't underdiagnose your patient, you will be less subject to review.

ISSUE	SUGGESTED SOLUTION
Treatment not commensurate with diagnosis. *Logical Treatment Program* *Supporting Evidence of Continuing Care* *Justifying Extended Care* *Status of Patient's Condition*	5. This can be indicated in the space allowed (#24D) on the universal claim form or superbill and on any reports. The acupuncturist must present and follow-through with a logical treatment program and show supporting evidence of continuing care. Adequate studies, planned reevaluations, and avoiding duplicating therapies are not only important but avoid a red flag by insurance companies. Use progress notes particularly to justify extended care. You can photocopy your daily treatment notes as required and with patient authorization, of course. Keep the insurer advised of changes in the status of the patient. Indicate on the universal claim form or superbill the date when the diagnosis is resolved and if there is any new diagnoses.
Fees not commensurate with treatment	6. Fees should be commensurate with treatment. Observe the best way to use procedure coding for the services you provide. Because codes have ceilings for insurance payment, coding may serve you better when you indicate a more complex CPT/RVS code with the reduced services modifier code --52.
Prognosis not commensurate with outcome of treatment	7. Show this in your reporting indicating the status of patient improvement. If there is any discrepancy, explain in writing. Provide second opinion if necessary. Back up with acupuncturist's progress notes and the patient's progress notes in litigation situations. Be careful in how you communicate the results

ISSUE	SUGGESTED SOLUTION
Results of Treatment	of your treatment—don't insinuate or promise a cure or imply your treatment is the only means of recovery.
Non-Commensurate Diagnosis, Treatment, Fees, and Prognosis	8. Use the 1) Initial Report and 2) Interim and Final Report forms in the forms packets to do insurance reports. They are standard report forms used in the health care professions with insurance companies.
Services involve conditions not considered treatable or not subject to favorable modification.	9. Use ICD-9-CM Code Book for correct diagnostic coding. If necessary send photocopy reference to similar case studies treated by acupuncture and modalities with favorable results.
Terminology	10. Use current medical terminology and the ICD-9-CM codes. Avoid using outdated or obscure terms which insurance companies won't understand.
Early Reporting	11. Submit your first report early in the course of treatment, particularly with workers' compensation cases.
Concise Recordkeeping	12. Be sure you itemize everything on the fee-communication slips so that it is reflected clearly on the patient's ledger, billing statement, and your reports.
Revealing the facts.	13. The acupuncturist and staff must be fair and in integrity. Does the patient have a preexisting injury, a re-injury or a new claim? Is the patient ready to be released from treatment?

ISSUE	SUGGESTED SOLUTION
Scope of Practice	14. Acupuncturists should be aware of staying within the scope of practice and billing for services inside of this scope. If a claim is denied on the basis of "beyond the scope of practice," send to the insurance company a photocopy of the Business and Professions Code section reference to "Scope of Practice for Acupuncturists" in your state."
Covered Provider	15. Quote sections appropriate from the Insurance Code in your state. Work with your local and state level organizations to effect legislation which will assure you will have rights to payment as a "covered" provider.
"Home of Plan" is other than your state and thus not subject to your state's insurance code requirements.	16. Quote your state law, if for your state it is contrary to your state law. Again, work with your local and state level organizations to effect change in law to protect both the patient, health care providers from insurance-backed laws which don't serve the public.
Insurance company takes stand that state law only applies to policies written after a specific date and that even though their plan may have been amended or renewed after that date, they are unaffected by the law.	17. Send a standard letter from the Department of Insurance of your state addressing this issue.
Plan is self-insured welfare benefit plan regulated by ERISA (federal government) and thus not subject to your state law.	18. U.S. Supreme Court case Metropolitan Life Insurance Co. v. Massachusetts, 105 S. Ct. 2380 (1985) can be used as state legal authority to support the fact that ERISA does not preempt state laws when the insurer is underwriting the risk (as opposed to solely administering the plan.

ISSUE	SUGGESTED SOLUTIONS
(Continued)	For purely self-insured plans, the Court in <u>Metropolitan Life v. Massachusetts</u> (op.cit.) held that certain ERISA plans were governed by applicable state law and that such state laws were not preempted by ERISA, thus showing that the ERISA preemption is not absolute. Also, the court held in <u>Rebaldo v. Cuomo</u>, 749 F. 2d 133 (1984) certain premises that the preemptive scope of ERISA is neither all-encompassing nor unlimited.

The most common causes for rejection of insurance claims come from paperwork problems. In many cases rejection is due to inaccurately filled out forms, sloppily-written bills, hazy or inaccurate diagnostic language and gaps in patient histories. No one problem in the clerical area seems more frequent than the others, so the best way to avoid rejection of claims and optimize your reimbursement is to follow directions exactly, be extra careful on diagnostic language and give a complete and accurate account of the treatment given.

There will be times when your careful monitoring shows claim problems that seem more difficult to resolve. The following chart may further help you determine what caused an incorrect payment so you can know to call the insurance company and fix the error.

COMMON PAYMENT ERRORS	WHY
Service is reduced.	The adjudicator may have downcoded the claim for lack of documentation.
Service is reduced.	The CPT code was converted to an RVS code that did not directly correlate with CPT.

Reimbursement is made at a much reduced rate.	Possibly a data entry error. Compare the CPT code submitted to the code paid.
Low reimbursement.	Precertification was not completed.
Low reimbursement.	Insufficient documentation to establish medical necessity. Provide further documentation.
Multiple units are paid as one unit.	The insurer "missed" your number in the units column.
The reimbursement for a procedure or service suddenly drops.	This could mean a recalculation of allowables or an error. Phone the payer.
Payment is not received.	Claim is lost or "caught in the system." Begin your inquiry.
Multiple procedures were not paid.	The insurance company either ignored the additional procedures or lumped them in with the primary procedure.

It takes the teamwork of you, your assistant, and the patient working together in your efforts to receive proper payment. You must do your part to be accurate. Be sure your patients and/or the insured fill in the "Verification of Insurance Coverage Form" and you keep a signed copy. If you are receiving "assignment of benefits," use the "Pre-authorization Form" to be given to the patient's insurance company if the insurance carrier requires Pre-authorization for service or treatment. Then be sure you have the insurance company's returned copy. This can save many insurance disputes later.

Because insurance involves so much processing and you are about the business of health care, let the patient handle their insurance responsibilities as much as possible. Using the "Patient Information on Insurance" form in the "*Insurance Forms Packet*" will help your patients to help themselves with their insurance. **Success with Insurance** will assist you to handle those insurances which you must handle completely.

How to Handle Reports

Keep report writing and typing time down to a minimum.

The report to have ready on the second visit for all new patients is the "Report of Findings" (See "Report of Findings" in either forms packets). Basic procedure is to have your assistant type the patient's name and complaints, the practitioner fills the remaining by hand. If you have a number of reports to handle, prioritize these reports on your desk with a deadline for completion.

Reports do not need to be elaborate or lengthy, and many computer programs are designed to be programmed to do fill-in the blank forms. Reporting can be done quickest from your computer patient profile or using the "Short Form Summary" (in the forms packets) if reports are expected each visit by the patient's insurance company.

If you don't have your patient profile on computer, use the patient's chart. Staff can fill in the basic patient information from the history/exam or progress notes forms and put that information on the report forms such as the Initial Report and Interim Report, and Workers' Compensation Billing and Report Form . For paid reporting use the "Initial Report Form". Record the following information: the patient's name, employer, date of injury of onset, circumstances of injury, patient's complaints, and the ICDA code numbers. Then you have to give your front-office assistant the additional information.

For the information on the reports which pertain to objective findings and examination, treatment, disability data, progress, and prognosis, and additional treatment needs, it is recommended that you use a dictaphone to dictate longer report information, so the office staff can type it onto the report. An acupuncturist would primarily use a dictaphone for accident and litigation cases where more extensive report writing is indicated.

The "Short Form Summary" is the simplest form to use to satisfy reporting needs to insurance companies. They can easily be set up on the chart with your fee slip. You do not have to automatically send longer reports to insurance companies unless it is specifically requested and required for payment. You do not have to send it if they are not willing to pay for it. However, you must get authorization for payment for each report before you send it, if you will be paid.

Workers' compensation reporting standards vary from state to state in the U.S. Workers' compensation requires acupuncturists who have legal primary physician status to fill out the "Doctor's First Report of Injury" and subsequently to use their forms for reporting. Other states have their own requirements for the type of reporting they desire. Check with your state workers' compensation boards for their current requirements.

What the workers' compensation companies want reported is the following information: the patient's name; their claim number, employer; date of injury onset; circumstances of injury and patient's complaints (in the initial report); the ICDA and generally RVS code numbers for billing; the date the employee's condition permits return to modified or regular work; when the employee's condition requires him or her to leave work; if and when you are planning hospitalization or surgery for the patient; when the employee's condition becomes permanent and stationary; when the employee's condition undergoes an unexpected significant change; when the employee is referred to another physician for consultation; or when the employer or workers' compensation company reasonably requests additional appropriate information.

Do not send reports to attorneys without first their authorization of payment for the report in writing. Payment for reports comes out of the attorney's fees paid for by the patient, and payment often comes directly out of the settlement. Getting authorization for payment of reports from insurance companies and attorneys may save you a lot of report writing, or at least allow you to be paid for writing them.

Court Preparation

Practitioners may end up in court either because the practitioner initiates the proceedings or because someone else, such as the patient, initiates the process. Usually the practitioner, who has primary responsibility for the care of the patient, will need to write a narrative report or more extensive yet, a deposition. If you are the acupuncturist working under supervision of a physician, you generally will not need to submit a medicolegal report or deposition. You may be requested to submit records. If you are the one initiating the proceedings, work with a good lawyer. It's a good idea to be building a good working relationship with a lawyer, in any case, because lawyers many times refer their clients to practitioners.

Make sure that you have your patient fill in the proper paperwork on the first visit. This includes: "Patient Introduction" (with consent to acupuncture treatment), "History Form," "Workers' Compensation Questionnaire" or "Accident Questionnaire" if work injury or accident, and liens, if authorized for treatment by the company, and the short form, "Patient Progress Report" on each visit. Have your patient sign a "Release for Medical Information and Authorization to Pay the Practitioner", if benefits shall be assigned to you, the acupuncturist. What patients say about their condition and progress plays a significant part in your conclusions. If you ever find yourself and the patient at odds in court, you have (his/her) handwritten records to show.

You may not actually have to appear in court. You would respond usually first to a subpoena for records, which would be handed to you before a court date. You may receive a phone call regarding the subpoena ahead of time, in which case the subpoena for records would be presented and an authorized person will appear to photocopy your records on the spot. Remember, a release of information must be signed by the patient before confidential information may be given. Check your records to be sure they are accurate, complete, comprehensive and intact. Your supporting evidence would normally include history and injury questionnaires, photocopied examination findings, patient and practitioner's progress notes photocopied from the patient's chart with initial and interim/final report and liens. For workers' compensation cases, include copies of the "Authorization to Treat" and the workers' compensation company own forms: "First Report of Injury" and liens which should have been sent to the workers' compensation company within the first ten days of treating. Their liens should be signed by you and the patient. This plus your billing is sufficient, unless a specific medicolegal report is requested.

A medicolegal report may be requested by the court or an attorney. It includes all of the information below:

- Patient's name, address, age, occupation, and marital status.
- Date and place of injury.
- What first-aid was rendered at the scene of the accident and who rendered it.
- Past history of the patient.
- Nature of injury and description of complications, if any.
- Findings of physical, neurological, and other examinations.
- Findings of auxiliary studies such as a doctor's X-ray or Kirlian photography and laboratory.
- Findings of subsequent examinations.
- Consultations.
- Diagnosis.
- Treatment.
- Follow-up visits.
- Prognosis and evaluation of permanent impairment.
- Concluding discussion & type of patient release.
- Acupuncturist's fee for services rendered and estimated fees for future services necessary.

You must have on hand, and file with the attorney, appropriate liens for payment, and a copy of all bills for patient services as well as for your medical report. The attorney is responsible for reimbursing the practitioner for his time in preparing reports, as well as for their comprehensiveness. Have the attorney sign the lien before you write or submit your report or medical information regarding the cost to the attorney and agreement by (him/her) that (he/she) will pay you for said charges. Charges are billed on a 99080 Code (as of this writing)and range from $25 for photocopied medical information to a broad range between $175-$800 for a medicolegal report. I have included a sample of a medicolegal report in the forms packets. If you prefer a more extensive model, I suggest you may want to purchase *The Medical Report Modular* on how to write a medicolegal narrative report, which can be obtained by writing renown insurance seminar leader, H.J. Ross & Co.26816 Vista Terrace, Lake Forest, CA 92630. The cost is approximately $35.00.

If you are called to court and cannot appear in court at the time and place designed by the subpoena, a deposition can be arranged with the attorney who served the subpoena. You will need legal papers for this.

You may be asked if you are covered by malpractice insurance. It is illegal to practice in certain states without it. In certain states, your license may be conditional upon receipt of malpractice insurance. You may need to show evidence of malpractice insurance coverage.

If you intend to go to court, make sure you consult with the supporting attorney ahead of time. The attorney will brief you on the kinds of questions which you will be asked. You will also discuss with the attorney what are usual practitioner fees for "expert" services. These fees vary from state to state and cover such things as courtroom appearance, travel time, time away from the office, meals, lodging, and miscellaneous expenses.

If you go to court, you will be required to bring to court complete records including films, and your bill for services rendered. In court you will identify yourself on the witness stand, answer questions regarding your credentials, and facts establishing your expertise. Speak in nontechnical language as much as possible. You will be asked to summarize the information in the medicolegal report. You will be asked what similar cases you have treated, to defend your diagnosis and prognosis, and your fees if they are not usual and customary for the area. Bring in any supporting evidence you can, including your staff in attendance on the case, if necessary.

Patient Management Procedure

Setting Time and Patient Care Management Patterns

A practitioner learns to develop a natural rhythm about the whole of his practice, as well as learns to develop a pace which serves one's patients the best. This pace is vital to the success of his practice because it shows where we give our attention, energy, and value and where we must adjust for practice success. Setting time allotments will focus your practice. For one, it can help your assistant to keep a patient flow rhythmical and prevent the "stacking up" syndrome which has created its share of many unhappy patients. A practitioner who cares <u>and</u> keeps an on time practice has the advantage.

Observe "how" the patient appointment book can be used. Not only is it used to schedule care, to establish a rhythm for the day, and keep your focus so the needs of patients are met with the greatest care and ease. It can tell you where control is being extended or is needed, what marketing and promotion measures should be taken, what hours should be extended or cut back, how to schedule paperwork around clusters of patient appointments, how to better organize the practice, and how the practice is expanding. The appointment record can give you valuable statistics such as the following: the number of patients scheduled, the number missed, appointments kept, call-ins and patients you've recalled, total visits, total new patients. Some appointment records have a space for recording the total business, total collections and the percentage of collections for the day and week. The practice management control forms to use with the schedule are:

> Daily Results: Practice Management Control Form #1
> Recalls for Rescheduling
> Re-Activation Program (used with recall procedure in **Volume II**)
> (These are in the *Big Forms Packet)*

When you have an assistant, make sure you receive a copy of the daily patient appointment schedule first thing in the morning. Consider your overall schedule for the week and how it fits together with your objectives. Once a week, make sure you review some basic statistics obtained from your patient schedule. This can bring up a lot of issues: hopes and dreams; fears and doubts; expectations and impatience; and what we want and what we don't want. However, remember: the statistics are management controls, which can show you what is happening and give you input so any necessary adjustments can be made.

The following page will help clarify what your weekly schedule looks like, how you will use your attention, and what you sense is the best time slotting for patient care. Volume II contains a weekly schedule and "to do list" to help you meet your goals and objectives.

Practice Hours

1. When do you focus on your practice? _____
   What days? _____
   What hours do you want to devote? _____

2. What time do you want to schedule your first patient?_____
   When don't you want to schedule a patient? _____

3. What time do you want to break for a meal? _____

4. What time do you want to return? _____

5. What time do you officially want to stop scheduling patients? _____
   What time do you want to close up daily?   _____
   What time do you want your last patient to leave?   _____

6. Often part of the assistant's job is the keep the practitioner account
   able for staying on schedule. This is particularly important to patient
   satisfaction. How will you handle keeping on time? _____

The Patient Schedule

Type of Patient	Type of Procedure	No. of Minutes
Established pt.	Regular Appointment	_____
Established Pt.	Re-Examination	_____
Established Pt.	Consultation	_____
New Patient	Consultaiton	_____
New Patient	First Exam/ Treatment	_____
New Patient	Report of Findings	_____
Established Pt.	Modality	_____
Established Pt	_____	_____
Potential Patient	Pre-consultation	_____
Work Injury -New	First Visit	_____
Auto, other Injury	First Visist	_____
Child	_____	_____
_____	_____	_____

Acupuncturist's Time Use

Activity	Hours/Week	% of Time
Working hours per week	_____	_____
Practice Planning Reviewing Daily, Weekly Schedule Reviewing Practice Management Controls	_____	_____
Staff Meeting	_____	_____
Patient Care (Treatment)	_____	_____
Case management -- Case planning, consultation, conferences with practitioners	_____	_____
Telephone and in-person calls	_____	_____
Public exposure -- Speaking engagements, seminars, advertising, practitioner/lawyer luncheons	_____	_____
Professional development - Association meetings, continuing education	_____	_____
Paperwork, reports, letters	_____	_____
No show or cancelled late appointments	_____	_____
"Days off", vacation time, including sick leave, other personal time _____	_____	_____
Regular Lunch	_____	_____
Total	_____	_____

4 Level Treatment and Home Care Recommendation System

The success of an acupuncture program is dependent 1) on diagnosis 2) treatment 3) patient orientation and education 3) the patient's attention to a consistent treatment schedule and 4) home care.

Set up your practice so that you offer at least four levels of treatment, and then **recommend** and **orient** patients to care beyond relief. A specific, consistent treatment schedule and follow-through on recommendations must be emphasized for positive results. A patient must also be assisted to realize the consequences to his/her own health by stopping or sliding on care. The four level approach is as follows:

1. **Intensified care** for symptom relief and pain control.

2. **Care beyond relief.**
   Eradication of tendencies causing the condition.

3. **Balanced optimum health care.**
   Rehabilitation. Elimination of root cause of the problem, if possible.

4. **Maintenance care.**
   Regular balancing / tuneups to keep in good health.

The success of the above four levels is magnified, by including1) home care recommendations, 2) do's and don'ts directions and recommendations, 3) report of findings, and a 4) planned re-evaluation visit. Patients must be informed that these "add to" and do <u>not</u> substitute for treatment.

By giving your patients the <u>best</u> of service, education and orientation towards greater options than just crisis relief, you serve your patients tremendously. Planned patient care = greater patient satisfaction with more lasting results in care = more enthusiastic patients who refer = practice growth, profit, and fulfillment.

If you use the "recommend one visit at a time" method with or without a plan regarding length of treatment or re-evaluation , you wil tend to build a <u>crisis care</u> practice, where patients are oriented to relief care. This does not provide the opportunity for patients to be educated into the three other levels of health care which provide their health with greater stability. Also from a business standpoint, the result   of one visit at a time practices is a higher practice turn-over which provides practice instability. Emphasis on health stability begets practice stability.

Setting Up Patient Visit Procedure
18 Ways to Increase Safe Practice Communication
--and Successful Practice

Good communication has many elements: trust, warmth, personable connection, concern. It is also a process of checking, verifying, and finding solutions such as a practitioner does to discern health, happiness, and well-being. "*Safe practice communication*" is specific. This is communication which is both verbal and written, insuring maximum understanding between practitioner and patient. Written communication is not only important because we live in a litigious society. It is important because our high health care standards expect practitioners to be thorough.

Practitioners can't be expected to communicate all procedural details with each patient verbally. However, certain kinds of communication should be in written form. Written materials are invaluable because they can be used for reference, can keep the practitioner and patient on track, reinforce new patient habit patterns and follow-through with home treatment. More often than not, they can assist you and your staff to avoid mistakes, misunderstandings, and liable suits.

Below are eighteen approaches with communication forms you can build into your practice for "safe practice." Select the approach and forms which fit for you to create *maximum* acupuncturist-patient communication in a *minimum* amount of time. The forms, mentioned here are in the *Big Forms Packet* of our Acupuncturist's Practice Management Guide Series. The procedures for implementing these approaches are further detailed in **Volume IV** for the practitioner and in **Volume II** for the front office assistant or practitioner.

1. **Make sure your qualification, services, and policies are clearly defined for your patient.** A "Welcome to Our Office Brochure" is excellent for this purpose.

2. **Educate the patient about acupuncture. Include what you do. It avoids misconceptions about what you do and don't do.**
   Give your patient a pamphlet such as "*Questions and Answers about Acupuncture*," its benefits, any hazards, and acupuncture for their specific condition. This should be done first. Then have him/her sign the statements

in the "Patient Introduction and Registration Forms" packet*— "Consent for Acupuncture Care", "Authorization to Treat" (if required by state), and "Release of Medical Information".

Fill a display rack with pamphlets in your reception room about conditions you (or acupuncture) treat(s) and how. Education increases your credibility, patient cooperation, and appropriate referral.

3. **Use clear concise means to determine if your services can benefit the patient at or before the consultation stage.**
Know initially what does and does not respond well to acupuncture care, as well as what signs indicate poor response to treatment.

In consultation, use the "Patient Introduction Sheet" listing their primary condition and conditions borderline or contraindicative to treatment as a starting point. If you want a better overview and want to conserve your time, make sure the patient fills out the history form for the consultation visit as well, so you get a quick overview. Don't start treatment with a patient or extend it if he should be referred out. This creates ill will, poor reputation, nonpayment, and can lead to claims suits. Utilize the most direct oriental medical methods of assessment either in consultation or later, in treatment.

4. **Let patients know what to expect regarding acupuncture care.**
Answer questions about acupuncture. Prepare them verbally for what it is to experience acupuncture care. Convey what patients can do to get the best results. Communicate the four basic options for treatment: 1) Intensified Care for symptom relief and pain control 2) Care beyond relief 3) Balanced optimum health care 4) Maintenance care and preventative care. Creating an opportunity for successful care in the patient's mind can be accomplished by using various timesaving and effective methods, such as audiovisuals, pamphlets, pre-consultation or post consultation briefing by staff.

5. **Document.**
Document what your patient's objectives are: what type of service he/she desires; how the patient classifies his/her condition; what his/her case history is; what the present concern is; and what the contributing factors are. It is helpful to know what kind of family support is available for the patient's healing. Use the "Consultation Form" and "History".

6. **Make sure you use both the appropriate means of patient assessment, and diagnosis within the scope of your practice.**
Use your own model of questions with your personal way of assessment.

* Pamphlets and forms available from Focus PM Pubs.

7. **Do an examination and record your subjective and objective examination.**
This provides a basis for determining treatment and recommendations. Use your own examination form. (This may also be called upon at any time by insurance companies or court.)

8. **Take the guesswork out of your patient's intentions.**
The shortest route to finding out where the patient stands with follow-through care is to ask and verify the patient's intentions. Notice the multiple choice questions: "What type of service do you desire?" and "How do you classify your condition?" These are on the "Patient Introduction Sheet," (page one of the "Patient Registration Form" in the *Big Forms Packet.*)

9. **Move along the following course in patient care planning:**
   1) Communicate what you can do to work with the patient successfully.[1]
   2) Focus on the patient's objectives.
   3) Reeducate the patient about the seriousness of the condition if in your judgment the patient is unaware of it.
   4) Focus on the implications of long or short term results regarding the desired result.
   5) Recommend with conviction.
   6) Agree on the length of service for the condition.
   7) Set the course in writing.
   8) Follow the plan.

   You can use your oral report of findings session to reeducate the patient as necessary in the four type of service options; gain agreement on recommendations; be clear on the patient's choice; and increase follow-through scheduling.

10. **Let patients know what to expect from your treatment plan.**
This can be done orally and strongly reinforced with written evaluation, recommendations, what to avoid, and confirming commitments. The following sheets were designed to minimize writing time, explanation time, and to convey a format for maximum results. The "Personal Acupuncture Report", with evaluation, schedule and recommendations set the course. "The Instructions for Care Sheet" and "Supplements Program," enhances it. "The Report of Findings and Health Care Proposal" creates a health care contract, if you choose to use this form. Follow-through is basically sticking to the plan and communicating patient need and progress.

---

1 Excellent sources of material on patient communication are acupuncturist Dr. Bradley Kuhns, Ph.D., C.A., originator of one of the first writings on neuro-linguistic programming called *Mind/Body Therapy: Visual, Auditory, Kinesthetic, an additional communication approach for the counselor,* and Bandler and Grinder's, *Frogs into Princes,* also a neuro-linguistic approach in communication.

11. Make it policy to give a written treatment plan handout to your patient.
It requires minimal writing, yet maximum benefit. It gives the patient something to which they may refer and continue to use. It also creates a sense of security, specific direction, and guidelines for their care. It documents your plan. Put the pages listed in #10 in a personalized folder to present to your patient.

12. Keep your Progress Notes on the patient.
They are a legal running record of your impressions and treatment. These are used as your reference and documentation for any reports required of you by an insurance company or in a litigation case.

13. Have the patient complete the short "Patient's Report of Progress" in the few minutes before each visit.
It insures a more concise and thorough communication from the patient to you. It also avoids misunderstandings or any misrepresentations later. Many patients forget to communicate important information when face to face with the practitioner, or remember only part of the information they intended to communicate. In these cases "The Patient's Progress Report" becomes invaluable.

14. Measure patient progress.
Patients want to know where they stand. Schedule a "reevaluation session" to assess the patient's progress within a *specific* period of time. Patients need progress marker points. Without them, they get discouraged and quit prematurely. The "Initial Report" or "Interim Reports" may be sent to a liaison practitioner at the time of reevaluation or as requested.

15. Plan for follow-through care.
Carry out the treatment plan schedule with advance multiple appointment scheduling, *including* the reevaluation date and time. Use a combination of the multiple appointment cards in the *Big Forms Packet*. It is vital that the front office personnel are clear on reasons for advance multiple appointment scheduling and the procedure to implement this (**In Volume II**). The advance scheduling multiple visit approach to follow-through care is to reinforce patient commitment to wellness.

Even if you are not sure how long a treatment plan will take, use the multiple appointment plan to build a commitment to the patient's desired end result, which is either intensified care for quick relief; beyond relief-- eradicating tendencies creating the condition; further series of care-- elimination of the root cause; and long range scheduling for preventative maintenance care.

16. Plan "consistency" into follow-through care.
    A. Use a good recall system. ((Use the Daily Results Form along with scheduling procedure in **Volume II**. If the patient calls, return calls promptly. Always and promptly reschedule cancellations or missed appointments.

    B. Reinforce keeping on their schedule, both with appointment cards and stating the time of appointment to your patient verbally. Use the specific dialogue in Volume II to handle excuses for missing appointments.

17. **Reinforce patient education on their health care, further support of the patient by family and friends, and benefits to others.**
    Suggest your new patients attend an "Orientation for Acupuncture Health Care Class" to help them understand your procedures, answer questions on how it can be applied, and reinforce their follow-through. Encourage them to invite their "support" person, family, and friends. The class will then familiarize a larger base of people with acupuncture health care's preventative, relief, and curative benefits. This can help promote referrals and other new patients as well.

18. **Get feedback on how your patients view their care, their recommendations, you, the staff, the service they receive.**
    Before the patient leaves the treatment room or the front desk, both you and your assistant individually should check to see if the patient feels "complete." Sometimes the patient will give a front or back office assistant feedback which the patient may not tell the practitioner, for whatever reason. Another way of getting feedback is to make a survey questionnaire available, which patients can fill out when they are waiting in your reception room. One is included in the Focus Practice Management's *Big Forms Packet* and in the 8 pamphlet series. This can give you valuable feedback on how patients perceive you.

Why the Safe Practice Communication Approach
Creates Successful Practice

These are the professional benefits and outcome:

- **Patient Results.**

- **Automatic Safeguard.**

- **Enthusiastic Patients and Referral.**

- **Freedom to Expand.**

- **Practice growth.**

Each of the safe practice procedures designed for patient-practitioner clarity and patient follow-through can be given a percentage value in practice growth. In a study which Dr. Fernandez completed, he found that exceptional practitioners who used the approaches and procedures listed below could expect larger percentages of practice growth increases. The procedures listed are the safe practice assets. They yield at least half of the results of his study.

ADAPTED PARTIAL LIST OF THE STUDY

Recommending the following type with commitment to service goals		195% [1]
Intensified Care --Quick Relief	25%	
Beyond Relief Program	100%	
Rehabilitation	40%	
Maintenance/Preventative Care	30%	
Pre-Report Tape or Audiovisuals		20%
Written Report of Findings		40%
Multiple Appointment Program		30%
Patient Reminder Cards Use		10%
Backsliding Prevention Program		40%
Patient Lectures		40%

The total of these together is a 375% increase in growth!

[1] Dr. Peter G. Fernandez. *Secrets of a Practice Management Consultant.*

What You Should Know about Records

Accurate records are essential with any practitioner-patient relationship. On the first visit, obtain information such as the patient's age, address and phone number, employment, employer, and insurance coverage. At this time the patient will write on the "Patient History Form" his/her chief complaint and health history. Make sure the history form is filled in completely. Proper consent and authorization forms must be signed. Remember, any case is liable to go to court, so maintain records bearing this also in mind.

The acupuncturist is responsible for accurate notes in relation to the patient's symptoms, complaints, and health history. Make sure the patient's chief complaint is written in exactly his/her own words. Keep an accurate record of each treatment, including dates, frequency, and what was done with that patient on each visit. One handy tool many practitioners use is color coding information: black pen for practitioner stated notes; blue pen for patient statements; red pen for spouse's comments. Attention to detail in record keeping benefits the practitioner and the patient. It assists the practitioner in giving the best possible care by carefully noting the treatment pattern and following and assessing the patient's response to treatment. It also can serve to protect the practitioner from malpractice.

Records legally should be kept at least seven years. Several factors should be considered in keeping the records even longer. Because many patients may be long term patients who are seen intermittently throughout the years, past history, though out of date, may prove useful. Also, it is important to remember that cases may go to court many years later, even after a person's death. Keep your records in a metal file cabinet that can be closed at the end of the day for protection from dust, fire, or catastrophe. Preserve your records as long as you can legally and comfortably do so.

A patient has the right to review his record, as well as the right to total confidentiality of his records. Before any records can be released to insurance companies or attorneys, or other physicians, for example, the patient must sign an authorization to release medical information. This release must be kept on file in your office. It is usually easiest to find if it is kept in the patient's file.

Although patients are entitled to have copies of their medical records via written request, the provider has the option to produce these within 15 days or prepare a detailed summary of the health records in place thereof. The patient therefore will not need to copy the medical records. Be sure you use consent and authorization forms. They are for:

- Malpractice protection
- Patient reimbursement for time loss from work.
- Income tax receipts and records for recommended equipment purchases.
- Verifying consent by parent regarding a child.
- Protecting the right of a patient.
- Protecting personnel of the clinic.
- Clearly stating "intention" on the part of the acupuncturist or the patient.
- Payment from an insurance company or legal case.

How to Reduces Malpractice Vulnerability

1. **Proper authorization to treat.**
   If your state or country requires that you have a signed physician referral, treat only after receiving signed proper authorization.

   Workers' compensation requires authorization from the company, employer, and in some states or countries, a physician referral as well. It does not mean you may provide services without signed authorization from a physician just because your state or country allows you to practice independently. If you treat workers' compensation cases, state workers' compensation and other workers' compensation companies may require a signed physician referral, even in states or countries which license acupuncturists as independent practitioners.

   Minors must also have signed parental consent before being treated.

   If you are in a state or country which requires supervision by a physician in order to practice, be sure you abide by the guidelines of your regulatory body regarding supervision requirements.

2. *Proper signed patient consent.*
   This applies to treatment or any new or unusual procedures, as is prudent. The Federal Food and Drug Administration requires acupuncturists in the U.S. to obtain a patient's signed informed consent for acupuncture care which states that acupuncture is considered experimental in the U.S. and that patients are aware of the risks as well as the benefits of acupuncture care.

3. **Have a check system for authorization, referral, and consent forms.**
   The acupuncturist's front office staff should be on the alert to make sure any state required physician referrals, consent forms, and authorization forms are filled in completely, signed properly, and on file before treating. Make it initial standard procedure to have all consent and authorization forms signed upon entrance and have a double check system for these forms before the patient leaves the office. A check mark on the ledger can indicate this. Note that verbal consent will not usually stand up in court.

4. **Patient Completed History.**
   Have your patients fill in a complete "History Form" and do so fully. A practitioner's intake form filled in by the acupuncturist is not sufficient to protect you in the invent of suit. Health care practitioners have been involved in court cases in which it is the patient's word against the practitioner's.

When the practitioner states the patient "denied having a condition" and/or "did not indicate a condition that could affect treatment and recommendations" on a history form," the history form filled out by the patient serves as proof in court— in the event of a suit. In cases where the patient says I had this condition, and the practitioner didn't check for it"--epilepsy, allergic reactions, etc.--and gave treatment or supplements counter-indicative, the practitioner has been held responsible --particularly in cases where a proper intake history was not taken by the practitioner and a patient history was not completed by the patient.

5. **Your history form should be designed to prevent and solve problems.**
   Check the design of the history form "used in your office. Sometimes acupuncturists get so busy in practice that they don't notice details which put themselves at risk unnecessarily, such as described above. Is your history form set up to obtain all the information an acupuncturist needs to check counter-indications, past or potential problems? Is the name and phone number of the patient's last physician on the form for consulting purposes? Is the history form specific enough? More general forms tend to provoke general patient response. Patients are often slightly amnesic in remembering health history, particularly negative health history. The more specific the history form, the more specific the patient response can be, and the more likely the acupuncturist can catch hidden problems.

6. **Control the appointment schedule.**
   The risk of grounds for malpractice are the greatest when the practitioner is rushed and overworked. Courts hold that the practitioner is expected to know his capacity and limits, and has no duty to attend to more patients than he/she can adequately care for properly. The practitioner must limit the number of patients he/she sees if volume adversely affects the quality of care. The front office assistant should be clear with the acupuncturist regarding proper time slotting for standard patient scheduling, and coordinate the scheduling of emergency patients or a patient load approaching higher than the practitioner's standard for the day. To avoid back up of scheduled patients and the pressure it creates on the practitioner, the assistant must be willing to call patients and adjust the schedule to work for everyone. Bad feelings with patients and the risk of errors and malpractice is highest when there is too tight of a schedule.

7. **Seek guidance when you are not clear.**
   "For whatever reason, the practitioner is obligated to call in a consultant whenever a case is beyond his or her experience or expectations. Document any further treatment when you refer a patient and coordinate with that practitioner."

Likewise, the assistant must be willing to consult with the practitioner whenever he or she is faced with a situation that is beyond his or her experience and skill. If any staff member is in doubt if something is appropriate, he/she should check with the acupuncturist.

8. **Advise carefully and within clear guidelines.**
Office staff should never offer suggestions to a patient, either in person or on the telephone, unless the practitioner has requested it. Even then, the acupuncturist's statements should be relayed precisely.

9. **Confidentiality.**
Remember that contact with any patient is a confidential communication unless a release of information is on hand.

10. **Clearly communicate your rationale for treatment and procedures.**
"Never let a patient be left with an impression that his condition has not been diagnosed or treated correctly." The front office assistant should treat every patient as if to prevent a potential malpractice case and should always provide assurance and support the clarity of the practitioner's rationale for treatment and procedures.

11. **"Make a clinical evaluation then treat according to acceptable procedures.**
Don't let the patient dictate treatment."

12. **Refer judiciously.**
Don't persist in treating a troublesome patient. Refer rather than practicing techniques beyond your scope of license. There are other disciplines which are licensed for those modalities. It's not worth jeopardizing your practice to save the patient a few dollars in going to another practitioner for a technique you know, but are not licensed to practice. Be aware of what equipment or therapies you can and cannot use.

13. **Use trained assistants only.**
Make sure your front office assistant and staff are clear on the safe practice guidelines and policies, that they have received proper training for their duties, and that those duties are clearly defined.

14. **Care with Clinic Records.**
"Be sure that all clinical records are neat, comprehensive, and up to date. Never make any alteration or use whiteout on the records, especially after a patient complains of injury."

15. **Progress Notes should be checked by the assistant for patient follow-through and completeness.**
"Progress Notes" should be date stamped by the front office assistant beforehand on the records and a record entered by the acupuncturist during each treatment. When each file comes back to the front office assistant, it should be checked to make sure a record is entered. If the assistant notes nothing was entered and the patient cancelled, she should write "cancellation" on the records, and record "rescheduled" and the date of reschedule in the space as soon as this is arranged.

16. **Prompt handling of patient calls and other follow-through on the part of both the acupuncturist and front office assistant is vital for proper care.**
Negligence can be proved if a patient or patient's relative calls, you fail to respond and provide adequate phone follow-up or follow-up care, and an adverse event occurs to the patient that would probably have been avoided by reasonable follow-up skill and care. ALWAYS return patient calls promptly and make sure that patients are recalled if they cancel or don't show. Make sure that patients are rescheduled or scheduled with a postcard reminder for maintenance care. Do multiple scheduling to promote follow-through care. Send maintenance check reminder cards out using a reminder card system. Don't unnecessarily drop or abandon your patients.

After the first visit, call the new patient later that day. Return your established patient's calls promptly. This says: "You care about follow-through and total patient care." Recalling patients can also trouble shoot patient dissatisfaction. It also promotes proper treatment plan rationale, as well as better patient communication.

Note that both insurance companies and courts observe the consistency of treatment provided by the practitioner, as well as the willingness of the patient and practitioner to stick to the treatment plan.

17. **Establish a working impression and diagnosis and record it.**
Have a clear rationale for your treatment and technique. Maintain good rapport and quality care.

18. **Complete recording on "Progress Notes" by the practitioner.**
"The patient's clinical records should contain a diagnosis which is supported by examination findings, examination and laboratory reports. Progress records should indicate both positive and negative symptoms. Progress notes should also support continuing care."

19. **Charge fees that are reasonable and customary in your area, and don't promise a cure.**

Make sure your fees are checked, and that they are reasonable and customary in your area. It's wise to do a fee survey. If you have a contract type of practice with payments in advance, don't imply promise of cure. Make clear agreements with your patients with planned reevaluation sessions. Give full value for your services.

20. **Correct film handling procedure.**

If you are an acupuncturist who is also an MD., DDS., or chiropractor, and you plan on x-ray films or Kirlian photographs, or feel they are advisable, it is recommended that films be interpreted prior to treatment. If you are responsible for taking the films, be sure they are made and processed correctly and that they are identified and filed correctly. Because it is not good policy to give films to patients, require a release from the patient so that the front office assistant can then mail the films to a referred practitioner. An increasing number of practitioners are also making a copy of all films released.

21. **Communicate your mutual responsibilities with patients, and have an agreement among staff regarding careful representation of the acupuncturist.**

Let patients know you are here to assist them in healing themselves, and discuss with them what their responsibilities are, as well as what yours are. "Both you and your staff should circumvent guaranteeing results or making extravagant claims in your enthusiasm for your skill and health care services. Only say to a patient what you would want repeated. Keep your communication simple and clear. Avoid what is called "snowing" the patient with double talk or technical jargon."

22. **Appropriate Witnessing.**

A front office assistant or other staff should be present in otherwise "compromising" situations. A female assistant or staff member can protect the practitioner by instructing all female patients in the proper method of wearing a gown, by properly draping a disrobed patient, by being present during an examination, and by being alert to passing remarks of a patient which may indicate the female patient's imaginary thoughts of the practitioner being "fresh."

23. **Impeccable needle sterilization procedure.**

If you sterilize your needles, monitor your equipment. It is recommend that a sterilization indicator be run through every sterilization cycle; and that regular, i.e., monthly or bimonthly, biological tests be run and records of the results be kept for an appropriate period of time. It is judicious to keep a written code of sterile procedures in your office and a log of sterilization dates.

Follow state guidelines meticulously for needle sterilization. The NCCA puts out a pamphlet on proper needle technique, which includes sterilization and storage procedure. We highly recommend following these guidelines.

AIDS is a real issue. *It's highly recommended that you use disposable needles.*

24. **Use disposable needles where appropriate and proper disposal procedure.**
This greatly reduces the question of transmission of possible AIDS from one patient to another. Avoid sticking yourself, particularly if you and/or your assistant remove. Set them down, and store them.

There are laws which regulate disposable needle procedure which state that disposable needles shall not be used more than once, and that all needles for disposal shall be placed in puncture resistant and leak proof hazardous waste containers. There may be questions as to where to incinerate these needles. There are companies which specifically provide the appropriate containers and provide special pick up of needle containers,which are taken to designated landfills or incineration facilities.

Most states and many countries regulate the type of storage, removal, and incineration procedure for needles. Aside from proper puncture proof containers, it is also advisable to use red garbage bags "marked" to indicate any other hazardous material to anyone else who would be hauling away or handling any dangerous or possibly contagious waste products.

25. **Proper and timely needle removal.**
Make sure all needles are removed before the patient leaves the treatment room unless appropriate otherwise. If needles are to be removed at a later date, have a system for follow-up, in case the patient misses the appointment for needle removal and the checkup.

26. **Observation of safety rules.**
"Your staff should always observe the safety rules stated by the manufacturer of health care equipment when administering adjunctive care under a licensed practitioner's supervision."

27. **Be aware of the legal limitations and protocols on the use of any medical device which is represented as "investigational" or "experimental".**
If you are thinking of purchasing a medical device, and are not sure it is

approved, you should contact the Department of Health Services in your state or country. Medical devices intended for use on humans must be approved by the Food and Drug Branch of the Department of Health Services before they are made available for general use by health care providers. A number of these devices may not be legally advertised, sold or administered within the state or country, even though the manufacturer claims the device is safe and effective. Unapproved use may be grounds for discipline by the practitioner's licensing board as unprofessional conduct and is regulated by the laws of a number of states and countries. There are provision by the states and many countries to investigate these new devices for future use.

28. **Care in handling patient injury.**
If a patient claims to your personnel that you, the acupuncturist has injured him/her, or that another staff member has injured him/her, you, as the acupuncturist must be informed immediately."

Give the appropriate care, get all of the facts, and reserve judgment. "It is important not to make or assume an outright admission of guilt. If someone is guilty of some serious error in judgment, statements should never be falsified. Receive proper counsel as necessary."

29. **When a patient threatens a suit, your first action should be to ask the patient to put (his/her) concern in writing to you.**
This is an excellent way for a patient to work through an emotionally charged issue. Professional mediation may be needed. Be sure the patient has signed a "Hold Harmless or Arbitration" clause before you treat. Let the patient know of your willingness to reconcile any problem with him/her. Generally you or your staff would not discuss the situation further until you contact an appropriate advisor. This could be a combination of any of these: counselor, attorney, or professional liability carrier. "Be cooperative but uninformative until proper counsel has been obtained."

30. **Improve your role.**
Attend those seminars and courses that are designed to improve your role as a capable practitioner or assistant . Current review gives a practitioner better control of his or her practice.

31. **Stay current regarding professional liability insurance.**
In states where there is no professional liability insurance, get involved in your association so that you can support obtaining it through your association. Insurance companies must be able to see acupuncture practitioners as taking an interest in and reaching towards higher standards of practice, including safe practice. Acupuncturists in those states and coun-

tries which currently have professional liability insurance cannot afford to take malpractice insurance for granted. Practice safely and for added protection, apply for malpractice insurance, know when your premiums are due and pay them on time. Continue to support the efforts of not only yourself, but the efforts of others, in achieving higher ethical and professional standards so that other states and other insurance companies will take an interest in covering acupuncturists as practitioners.

32. Be current with acupuncture law and practice within the scope of your license.

Have an awareness of current acupuncture law so you can be aware of what is appropriate legally, as well as morally. States within the U.S., as well as other countries, vary in their definition of scope of practice. They vary in the degree of independence they allow an acupuncturist and in the types of techniques, modalities, equipment, and supplements (food and drug) which can be given and/or used.

Individual responsibility for safe practice and a unified effort towards higher standards can only affect the public view of acupuncture in a more positive manner. You are greatly honored for doing your part in achieving this.

Note: Focus Practice Management Publications' *Big Forms Packet* contains forms which are specifically designed and essential for safe practice. Quotes are from "Malpractice Considerations", _Chiropractic Paraprofessional Manual_, Practice Administration and Management, American Chiropractic Association, c.1978. The Acupuncturist's Business Management Guide: Safe Practice Guidelines and Policies, c.1986, 1987, 1988, by Cynthia Flint Bestani, ISBN :0-944876-23-4

Telephone Procedure and Scheduling

Telephone dialogue, procedure, and policy must be handled carefully because the telephone is one of the first contacts that most patients will have with you and your staff, and the value of a good first impression is immeasurable. The objective of good telephone procedure is to motivate even casual callers to become healthy patients through the service of your office.

The telephone is the mechanism of transmitting not only voice, by the representation of your practice. Attitude, personality, and manner of the one who answer your phone creates a practice image in the mind of the patient and a feeling impression about your practice. This is one reason the ability to handle public relations by phone is so important. Who you hire to handle your phone should represent a profession which has the proven ability to get sick people well, and provide a link of service to connect both acupuncturist and caller.

How the telephone is handled in your office:
■ Can inspire or detract potential patients.
■ Can bridge the barrier between the unknown and the known for inquiring patients.
■ Can help people quality themselves for care.
■ Can help justify the cost of care.
■ Can affect the kind of scheduling changes which are made.
■ Can provide backsliding prevention by specific dialogue.
■ Can motivate patients to follow-through on scheduling care.
■ Can help motivate patients to pay for past due services.
■ Can assist people to get through objections to handling finances.
■ Can communicate how your practice benefits your patients.
■ Can communicate to enhance healing.
■ Can help clarify issues with insurance companies and help you get paid for your services.
■ Can set good or poor protocol between practitioners in the same office.
■ Can affect the handling of emergencies.
■ Can affect the way messages are handled.
■ Can dramatically affect your practice reputation and image.

The protocol, dialogues and procedures regarding each one of the above is contained in *Volume II.* Your staff as well as yourself will benefit by learning the dialogues and procedures as they are presented in *"The Front Office Training and Reference Manual."*

The front office assistant should personally handle all telephone calls whenever possible because he/she can praise you and acupuncture with an emphasis that is not possible for you to do as the acupuncturist yourself.

Since the front office staff answers the telephone 95% of the time, he/she is best in position to make your office and its services sound inviting to both the prospective patient and the established patient. This is an essential part of a staff's service.

Scheduling

Like creative visualization, scheduling is an art. You want the one who does your scheduling to be your personal representative. You wouldn't want to settle for less. It is worth hiring someone who can believe in you, who loves public relations, and is detail oriented enough to handle the specifics of running an office. It is also important for that person to have the best training.

Volume II goes into detail on setting up the appointment book, how to record in the book, and contains a sheet for setting up your time allotments for different types of patients. It sets the foundation for scheduling procedure, including dialogues and procedures for how to schedule an inquiring patient or a workers' compensation and personal injury patient, how to schedule multiple visit appointments, when to do recalls and how to handle backsliding prevention scheduling.

The secret of carrying out effective scheduling is hiring and training the right person, who understands the goals and objectives of scheduling, and is committed to carrying those out.

It comes down to the following: The intention of continuing care scheduling is to get patients to come regularly until they are well, and to create a commitment to follow-through on a recommended program. The aim is to provide quality care and inspire enthusiasm so they will, in turn, naturally become lifelong referral-type patients. The desired result: Building and maintaining a steady and healthy referral practice.

How will you set up your telephone procedure and scheduling and train personnel? _____
_____

How to Assure Follow -Through Care

Patient Recalls and "Backsliding Prevention" Scheduling

90% of patients who cancel and are not followed up by the practitioner's office, will stop care prematurely. This jeopardizes both, the patient and the practitioner.

Recalls are calls returned to patients who have called and left messages and requests a return call; or have cancelled or missed an appointment with or without phoning. Backsliding prevention scheduling is an art which requires a conviction in what you as the practitioner are offering the patient, provides dialogue which removes barriers to treatment, and reinforces the patients commitment to treatment and cure.

Three things for a practitioner to notice about patient recall and backsliding prevention procedure:

1. Properly carried out these two procedures prevent both poor patient-practitioner-staff rapport, prevent patients prematurely quitting treatment, prevent erratic treatment and follow-through of recommendations, and can prevent negative or neutral practice image and reputation.

2. These procedures should be built into your practice as early as possible. The longer a practitioner waits to correct patient backsliding the more damage it does to a practice. Patient recall and backsliding prevention procedure is clearly addressed step-by step with phone dialogues in *Volume II.*

3. Because proper patient care is at stake, your reputation is at stake, and your practice growth is at stake, your care and selection of your front office person who handles these two procedures can greatly contribute to your practice success or your failure.

What you can do is to be sure your front office assistant learns the procedures, understands the importance behind them, and carries them out effectively. Share the "10 Good Reasons for multiple visit appointments with your front office assistant." Discuss your procedures in your office meetings and manage by an approach called walking around management. When you listen to the way he/she handles these procedures on the phone and he or she is excellent at these two procedures -- which Dr. Fernandez attributes 40% in practice growth -- reward your assistant for a job well done.

Part of total patient care, including a maintenance program, is both long term and short term follow-up . You can do your part by making sure the patient always leaves with a follow-up appointment time-- even if it is a 6 month check. Some offices make it policy that a patient never leaves an office without an appointment or having the patient sign a reminder card for maintenance care checks. This does not mean prolonging any unnecessary care. We are talking about ethical care. Never drop your patients. Look at yourself as "their preferred life long practitioner." Wish them well when they complete a cycle of care. Support their follow-up health maintenance care, referral, and returning when any other conditions return.

Use all the reinforcers possible for communicating with the front office person when the patient's next scheduled appointment is. What are the reinforcers? Tell the patient when the next appointment time should be, verbally tell your front office assistant, and use a fee - appointment slip[1] that goes to the treatment room with the patient and comes back out to the assistant at the front desk before the patient leaves.[1]

10 Good Reasons to Schedule Multiple Appointments

From the standpoint of patient care and follow-through planning, consider this: Scheduling multiple visit appointments with a planned reevaluation time greatly enhances practitioner acceptance, his/her recommendations, and patient cooperation to achieve desired results.

Multiple visit appointments set, build, and provide:

1. **The Patient's Orientation toward Planning.**
   If you use a multiple appointment approach, which means that you schedule a series of appointments at one time, your patients will most

---

[1](The fee, communication-appointment slips are in **Volume II** with an explanation for use.)

likely schedule their lives around the existing appointments. If you schedule appointments on a visit by visit basis, these appointments will be scheduled around the rest of their lives. This helps the patient by building consistency in treatment and a greater probability of increasing satisfying treatment results. It provides greater stability for the patient and for the practice with greater follow-through.

2. **A more Realistic Approach to patient expectations about health care.**

   Multiple visits can serve those patients who have unrealistic expectations, who came expecting an instant cure of certain immediate results. It can assist those patients to not stop care prematurely. Expectations can be more realistically handled by working towards a health care goal within a specific time frame.

3. **Patient Security and Continuity.**

   It can give worrisome or anxious patients a sense of security and continuity -- a sense of their care being followed. If the patient becomes worrisome or anxious over treatment, he/she is more likely to call or come and discuss care at the next appointment, or make an earlier appointment, rather than quitting prematurely.

4. **Patient Assurance of consistent patient care and reinforced repatterning.**

   Patients know (or soon discover) they can get consistent attention and reinforcement, rhythm and a new pattern in their life to achieve their health care needs and objectives.

5. **Patient Orientation.**

   It gives the patients a time to be oriented and be educated regarding the benefits of their acupuncture care, and to learn more about their care so they can cooperate more with their treatment program. The added "Patient Orientation Health Care" class(es) is an extra plus for many patients. Many patients don't really want a hit and miss approach to achieving their needs if they can see the rationale for meeting short or long range objective.

6. **Patient Acceptance of Needed Services.**

   It provides an opportunity to give the patient further education and motivation for additional *needed* services. Sometimes the patient won't see the need to go beyond temporary relief until after the first one or two treatments. It gives patients a chance to experience progress from temporary relief, to the eradication of tendencies causing the condition, to removing the cause of a condition, to a maintenance program.

7. **Clearer Comparison and Reevaluation of Initial Condition, further Conditions, and Progress.**
Multiple visits provide a greater comparison and reevaluation of the patient. Sometimes the original symptoms (conditions, attitudes) may be exaggerated on the initial visit, symptoms may shift, etc. From the patient standpoint, patients like to see a progress point in time. Multiple visit appointments with a reevaluation date serves that purpose.

8. **Monitoring, Input, and Feedback.**
It provides the patient consistent monitoring and encouragement to follow-through home care recommendations and gives you further opportunity to offer suggestions and input to benefit the patient.

9. **Good and Lasting Personal Rapport.**
You get to know the patient on a personal basis. The patient may have the benefits of many "extras" which add to their well-being and enthusiasm about life, you and your practice. Their enthusiasm about your extra care can begets life long returning patients and referrals.

Patients who have good communication with their practitioners, who recognize the extra effort, who have been on a set program tend to be happier with the results and more willing to not only refer, but pay.

10. **Complete Services.**
Multiple visit appointments offer greater options than just relief. This has many ramifications discussed in the section entitled, "4 Levels of Treatment and Home Care Recommendations."

Multiple visit appointments allow you to plan for patient care, your schedule, and for consistent revenues and expansion. Multiple scheduling, according to Dr. Fernandez, accounts for 40% of practice growth.

Referral Planning

Referrals occur because people receive a favorable impression of you, feel grateful, and acknowledge you as their healing link. It also means reminding to your current patients that they are the link for other people to get well too. Appeal to this fact. Since practitioners depend on their patient base for 75% of their referrals, why make it a secret? Tell people you depend on them for referrals. It's that simple! Timing is important, of course. Once you've found a referral source, the key to success is to act. These are examples of acts that will achieve your objectives:

1. Schedule and/or encourage all new patients for a one time "Initial In-Office Orientation Health Care Class" for acupuncture patients. Invite them to bring their support person and friends who want to know more about acupuncture health care.

2. If a patient mentions the name of a friend who he feels could be assisted, be genuine in your concern, and ask him to bring (friend's name) in with him on his next visit and schedule both together.

3. Give and display reception room pamphlets on specific conditions and how acupuncture works. Give a pamphlet to patients who have the condition and ask them to read it thoroughly. You or your assistant should ask if he has a friend for whom it would be appropriate. Follow-up. Even though we may be treating the whole person, and not just symptoms, pamphlets on conditions do get patients' attention.

4. Give and display "We Love Referrals" referral pamphlet and "Courtesy Consultation" cards, (in Big Forms Packet) and give it to patients who begin to express enthusiasm. Let them know how much you appreciate their referrals

5. Provide patient incentives for referral: A free treatment or special gift as a thank you for each referral works!

6. Educate your patients about further benefits of acupuncture. They will quote you. Give them pamphlets on acupuncture for specific conditions. If they are enthusiastic about your services, they will refer to anything you say or read and share with others what you give them, particularly if they see results.

7. Patient appreciation for referral goes a long way. The Patient Letter; Acknowledgment letter for referral; bulletin board acknowledgment of patients who have referred, the "We Love Referral Pamphlet" — all tell patients how important referral is to you and how much you appreciate their referral.

With referrals in your practice, you must do three very specific things.

1) Earn your patient's loyalty. Create loyalty and enthusiasm.

2) Use to advantage specific referral-building tools to remind patients to come to you and follow-up.

3) Have your receptionist make referral building and follow-up procedure part of her every day job.

In order for your referrals to grow, you can structure what you will do to create loyal referrers. Referrals do not happen without thought. It is vital not only to the survival of your practice, but to its expansion. How far do you want to go to reach those who can most benefit from your services?

A sample "Referral Plan" might follow this outline:
(This goes hand in hand with the patient care plan which you create.)

Visit 1:   **Establish referral leads.**
Ask by whom were you referred?
Who is the referring physician? Get written authorization to call.
Note to follow-up before visit 2. Schedule call to physician.
Check history of health problems of family.

Provide patient assurance and establish availability.
Give your home number to the patient in case of emergency, or problem.
Do follow-up evening phone call to new patient in pain.
Change a home remedy, night position in bed, breathing exercise.

Visit 2:   **Report of Findings, Recommendations, Directions for care**
Clarification of type of care — relief, stabilization, optimal, maintenance, prevention.
Touch and Tell Procedure
Be sure the patient was aware of a change in experience.

Establish consistency, quality, and safe referral.
Statement: "Each of my patients gets an individualized health care plan."

Visit 3: **Reinforce follow-through and strengthen faith.**
Check follow-through on recommendations.
Law of Similars: "I had great success working with a patient with this same condition, (stress what happened, and how she followed through with treatment.) _____ is one of my best patients."

Visit 4: **Schedule health care class appointment seat(s).**
"Bring the person who can support you most with your health care to the class."

Visit 5: **Schedule health care class seat(s).**
Thank the person for referring.

Visit 6: **Drop seeds:**
Refer to people who you cared for with conditions such as allergies or colds. Relate it to seasonal care.

Visit 7: **Reevaluation Visit.**
Assess progress. Schedule a new series if needed.

Visit 8: **Give the patient a pamphlet for a person with medical problems they know.** Use your power of authority to motivate. "Bring their friend or relation in."

Visit 9: **Bring up your specialty.**

Visit 10: **Bring up a patient (not by name) whose progress excites you.**
"We depend on our patient for referrals." Recommend the *"We Love Referrals"* pamphlet.

It usually takes at least four educational suggestions for a referral to occur. If your assistant does backup help with referrals, they will most likely occur faster. The first series of visits are oriented more toward relief care. The next series goes beyond relief care toward stabilization. Patient enthusiasm and loyalty grows, and referral-building is appropriate at this time. The next series is oriented to optimum results and patient education. Patients are then guided towards prevention and maintenance. Patient loyalty is strengthened with a caring attitude and a planned program geared to successful results. Most who experience this will become long term-referring patients.

Volume IV: Patient Communication, Public Relations and Marketing goes into more specific planned referral building procedure for practitioners, as well as has numerous examples of marketing, and same advertising related to this section.) **Volume II** is specifically detailed for front office procedure referral building procedure.

PERSONNEL--YOUR INVALUABLE SUPPORT

The Case for Hiring Good Staff

Successful practices are collective team efforts. Other than your own vision, energy, healing abilities, and administrative capability, productive employees are the backbone of a practice. Their abilities can either make or break a practice. They are one of the two key important assets of a practice.

So often inexperienced practitioners tend to recruit and pay at lower levels than they should and are slow to recognize what creates quality in their practice. They only gradually upgrade their practice and their staff as they come to value the contributions of truly productive employees. The pitfall of hiring cheap staff at first occurs often because a practitioner imagines that he/she can do all the important work him/herself. Mostly however, the tendency is to underestimate the make-a-difference contributions of good employees. They are often, as it turns out, foolishly cost-conscious. They hope to "get by" with very ordinary employees.

Another pitfall of practitioners who hire ordinary staff is that they either invest available funds in less productive areas or else distribute them to themselves. Although their overall goal may be "cost-effectiveness care, they overemphasize the "costs" of a good staff at the expense of "effectiveness." Cutting corners on staff costs is a false economy that, in the end, undercuts effectiveness. Poor staffing also occurs when a practitioner hasn't adequately identified the needs of the practice and matched those needs with the person who could best support them to have the vision for their practice.

How does an unmotivated ordinary employee undo a good practice? This kind of employee doesn't enliven a practice with enthusiasm; he/she may even turn patients off by subtle indifference; He/she doesn't put in the extra to inspire a potential patient to make the appointment. He/she isn't always conscientious about scheduling patients before they leave, nor doing backsliding prevention. He/she does not ask for referrals or make the effort to point to benefits of care. He/she may not feel compelled to return phone calls, may over-book the schedule without seeing how he/she created the consequences, and can be lackadaisical about financial communications. A practitioner not only loses patient enthusiasm and ensuing referrals. The acupuncturist's practice's reputation may insidiously suffer with such an employee. Any efforts by the practitioner to build his/her practice is counteracted. So remember that your practice is in good part the sum of the work of your staff.

You alone may be responsible for hiring and managing the staff. You also are responsibility for making sure that you find and keep employees who carry out your objectives and are good managers of your practice.

First rate employees fill the gaps in your own experience, interests, and skills. They allow you to concentrate on excellent patient care and treatment, to do what you do best, and handle the other administrative things which only you can do.

If you hire good employees, you don't have to monitor their work as carefully, redo what they have done, or clean up the mess afterwards. Good employees plus specific practice management control procedures can free you from damage control. Good employees can save you valuable time, energy, and money.

Good employees set an example of the kind of care and business you want to promote. When patients first call, 95% of the time their first impression of you is from your front assistant. This should be a link which conveys faith in you, confidence in your procedures, and appreciation for the patient. This attitude should be reinforced from the time the patient first walks through your doors to when he/she leaves.

One of the most important assets, not often recognized at first is the value of an employee who has the ability to promote sincere rapport, educated procedure, good referrals, and the "extras" with care. If you hired someone who was efficient but did not have this dedication to rapport building, your practice would suffer in reputation. On the other hand, if your staff is so people oriented, they don't keep the practice on track, you are in trouble too. Good employees who go the extra mile, think carefully and establish good patient relationships, more than make up their salaries in the profits you receive.

Does the patient pick up sincere interest and care from your employees? Do they get the extra attention to detail that makes your practice unique? Do your employees provide encouragement? Do they give more than expected? Do they put themselves in their patients shoes?

Are the patients first in the practice? Do they give your patients the "extra" attention which creates enthusiastic patients? Do they know how to icebreak an uncomfortable situation? Do they serve people while handling money? Do they communicate with patients about the benefits of acupuncture care and promote you, your educational materials, and health care classes with patients?

Good employees create energetic work environments which promote high morale, integrity, and encourage more effective participation. They are the ones who can follow good team objectives which make you say "Yes!" to these questions: Do they find ways to easily ask for referrals? Can they troubleshoot? Do they promote safe practice? Do they add to your office efficiency, procedure and care? Do they study office procedure and routine? Are they alert and take action when inertia begins to set in? Do they give thought to a better, simpler faster way of doing what they do that would save time, energy, and money or get a better result? Do they set an example for your patients' being on time and in synchronicity by being on time themselves? When a new procedure or technique is introduced, do they cooperate willingly? Do they have good communication with you? Do they have infinite faith in you? Have they made your vision for your practice part of their own? Do they have the "WE" spirit?

All of this may seem obvious. However, it nonetheless has taken many practitioners years to appreciate hiring good staff. The lesson learned is "Don't cut corners of the staffing. Hire good people and make sure you spend productive time developing them."

Certainly you put a large investment of time, energy, and money in the training of your staff. It is well worth taking sufficient time to find the qualities you want in the ones to surround you, to take care of you, to run the day to day details of your practice, to care for your patients, and to serve together with you in mutual respect and fulfillment.

The Keys for Good Teamwork

1. Decide what your objectives are, the specific job needs of the practice, and the results you expect form staff. Using a staff policy.

2. Hire employees so you match their talents , attitude, experience, and objectives with yours. Do they complement?

3. Have clear job description as well as use a procedure manual. Set clear top priorities. Clearly communicate what needs to be done, and by whom, and how they keep track of their results.

4. Effectively delegate substantial authority to strong dedicated employees and contractors, such as accountants, financial planners, who monitor your practice and give you feedback.

5. Manage the need to please / avoid conflict, your self-esteem, and need for control. Honesty with sensitivity works well between people.

6. Using management control forms* to aid staff in keeping track of their results and for practice review; holding staff meetings regularly to inspire team spirit ; getting staff feedback, and making any adjustments for practice progress.

7. Use management control forms (in the *Big Forms Packet)* to aid staff in
    keeping track of their results and for practice review. Hold staff meetings regularly to inspire team spirit. Get staff feedback, and make any adjustments for practice progress.

8. Appreciate your employees so they feel good about themselves, the objectives they achieve, and the job they perform. Providing job satisfaction and job enrichment incentives.

Why Do Practitioners Have Problems with Delegating?

Delegating doesn't seem to come naturally to most people, let alone most practitioners. It is something which is learned as a necessity, so that a practice can function without undue stress, and profit without undue problems.

Practitioners who can't or don't delegate either have a very small practice , many times limiting their ability to grow, or else their practices grow, but they grow chaotically and progressively develop one problem area after another.

Many practices start out as a husband wife team, where the wife is the front office assistant. By aiding her husband in starting practice, she is establishing both her husband's and her life-style for the rest of her life. She has chosen to marry a man with a purpose, and she is able to share in this. Often a wife assists in the beginning to help her husband reduce the overhead. If the wife is a natural promotor and takes it upon herself to understand all aspects of practice management, a husband and wife team can create a highly successful practice. Unfortunately, most practitioner's wives are not always strong in the kind of promotional and collection skills necessary to expand a practice. It is often a sensitive subject to ask a wife to take a different role with the practice and hire a stronger front office assistant, particularly in families where family loyalty is very strong. The desire to "not rock the boat" has caused numerous practice to struggle along and in some cases fail.

If you don't delegate to effective family members or personnel, you become either a prisoner of detail and work overload, or you take care of patients and let your practice as a business slide, including the paperwork, missed appointments, lost referral opportunities, and problems. You also will have no free time to observe, reflect, and plan. Any personnel or family member you had hired to do what you hoped they would, will in time hand all their decisions and problems over to you. You either will end up doing part of other's work, let it slide, or end up doing it poorly.

Sooner or later, if your practice grows beyond the embryo size, you must:

1. Accept the need for reorganization and some specialization
2. Spend some time considering the most effective way of carrying out your objectives.
3. Reconsider who and how you delegate what you or your family members formerly assumed.

It is effective staffing, delegating, as well as marketing, which will allow you to concentrate your time and energies where they count most and to expand your practice.

If the principles and importance of delegation are so obvious and compelling, why do so many practitioners fail to delegate or do it so halfheartedly? **Clearly, it is difficult to share responsibility, have others meet your standards, or adjust responsibility because of affiliation issues, self-esteem issues, and control issues which arise.**

Not only has it been difficult to ask a family member to change roles in the practice. Many practitioners simply have difficulty with the idea of changing anything because it might generate conflict, disharmony, or upset the status quo. The unwillingness to redefine the practice needs, to rock the boat with staff for fear of hurt feelings, or deal with practice problems, has killed countless practices. These are the practitioners who allow "their need to please" to take control over good business sense. These practitioners find it difficult to ask staff or family members to do things differently, to tell staff what they don't want, to let the "ordinary non-motivated" staff go after the trial period is up, and shy away from hiring again. Altruistic motivation, when it continuously overrules practicality in a practice, turns the practice into a philanthropy. The practice no longer remains a profit generating business, either struggles, or fails in the end.

Regarding control issues, a number of practitioners become preoccupied with control and perfectionism. They over protect their practices as if it was a baby or little child. They feel acutely uncomfortable and even remiss in relinquishing authority to anyone else, or in the case of husband-wife teams, anyone outside of the family. However, the time does come in growth when a practitioner has to prune his or her activities and recognizes that others can handle the everyday practice management better than the practitioner and employed family members.

Regarding both esteem and control issues, another comment that is often made is, "It's difficult to keep your fingers out of things you did as you built the practice." Others feel they'd like to delegate more, but feel

there staff just isn't up to it. They feel they'd better do it themselves."
Sometimes there is an attitude that no one can handle the practice better
than the practitioner and his/her family. Often a practitioner has never
really attempted to delegate or has done it poorly. Maybe he expects more
of an employee than he does of himself and is intolerant of anyone's
performance except his own or his family members.

Another problem practitioners have in delegating is that they find
it difficult to make the shift from the details of daily operational tasks to
one of simplifying their role -- i.e. treating patients, supervising activities,
handling necessary callbacks, writing reports, and timely practice review.
If a practitioner is to be freed up to practice and overview it, he/she must
hire and delegate authority over operations. It's a matter of redefining
one's role as both administrative and practicing acupuncturist, instead of
everyday operations performer. He must focus on achieving the long
range objectives of the practice. He then uses a daily log, sticks to a
schedule, works his/her plan, and manages staff.

Another group of practitioners find it difficult to deal with business
and want to delegate it all and be rid of handling business. These
practitioners should delegate as much as they can. *However*, staff must
be given clear objectives, know who handles what responsibilities, and
what the top priorities are. The practitioner must still monitor his/her
practice, get or give feedback give well earned appreciation to staff, or
adjust the practice based on feedback controls.

The practitioner at some point must be willing to look at *whatever*
the needs of delegating are and take an honest look at the whole practice
--both its successes and failures. In redefining the practitioner's role as
administrator and healer, the questions to ask are: "What kind of *support*
do I and the practice need to meet my objectives? What are the guidelines?
What are the priorities? What kind of delegating will support this?   How
will I communicate this?" (We'll be discussing this in upcoming sections
of Vol I & Vol II.).

Good patient and practice procedure includes not only setting and
communicating your priorities and getting, giving, and receiving feedback; but hiring those who do likewise. Then the practice can grow
successfully.

Effectively delegating may be one of the practitioners' biggest
issues in which to come to terms. If we are to be effective healers with

others in healing the fragmented self not just in body, but with mind/ emotions, and spirit, it must begin with ourselves. Identifying the issues is the starting point. It takes real honesty to face these issues. How do the issues spoken of here relate to you? Take this into meditation.

How do you feel about delegating? _____
_____
What may be preventing you from delegating?_____
_____
_____

What may be preventing your from delegating more effectively? _____
_____
_____

Does that need to be so? _____What new choices can be made about that?
_____
_____

*..to grow successfully, profitably, is to both delegate
and communicate effectively.*

Effective Delegation

Part of developing good staffing and good delegating is giving employees a clear job description of responsibilities so it is obvious *who* will handle *what* responsibilities. The second part, so often missed, is giving an employee a clear idea of your objectives and priorities in carrying out their responsibilities! The third part is giving the personnel room to carry out your objectives, giving them the built in control forms and procedures to help them be accountable for the results they produce. The fourth part is giving them incentives and rewards for good results.

Everyone needs to know what is expected and what is top priority. Many employees know their responsibilities well. However, they don't always know the objectives and priorities for carrying out their job. Your staff must be clear on both theirs and yours. If your staff catches your philosophy that they can grow individually through the growth of the practice, they will support your practice. If you communicate your practice from your desire to promote team objectives, you will create a more cohesive team spirit which will give added value to your employee(s)' responsibilities and everyone's good.

You will need to decide how many hours a day you need assistance, what you need help with, and the best way of fulfilling the need so that the practice and you are freed up to expand.

Many of your services will be handled in the office. Perhaps some of your needs can be handled by contractors outside your practice, such as billing by medical billing service; Insurance handling can be supplemented by a part-time insurance clerk. An answering service or answering machine can handle phone messages when your assistant is unavailable. A part time or full-time secretary could be hired and shared by everyone in your practice. An existing employee could be paid extra hours to do overload typing. An accountant or outside bookkeeping can handle your expense recording.

You will have to determine your trade-offs when you hire, and take great care when you delegate. Relevance of personal experience have to be weighed against character, resourcefulness, human relations skills. Front office skills require the above. Maturity, reliability, exactitude are important in bookkeeper and accountant positions. Background and experience are important when hiring an insurance clerk. When hiring part-time insurance clerks, you would want someone who had experience with insurance already in the medical field. Experienced technical part-timers or full-timers can often take greater responsibility for correct procedures. When making hiring decisions, look for dedication and resourcefulness and weigh those against lack of experience.

Weigh the importance of good communication. If you practice in the United States, for example, and English is not your first language, hire an assistant 1) who speaks your language,. 2) communicates well in English, and 3) has the abilities we discussed. This kind of assistant is worth his weight in gold.

(See Delegating, Hiring and Staff Decisions Questionnaire, and the Controlling and Delegating Aptitude and Next Steps Questionnaire)

How to Set Your Staffing Foundation

Effective practices invest the time and effort by being thorough in their hiring process. We have included a section on the "Hiring Process" to help you with your hiring procedures. The *Big Forms Packet* contains the necessary forms to assist with hiring as well.

Effective practices then develop clearly defined office policies and personnel procedures that cover all employee questions and concerns. This includes checks and balances which prevent abuse of the system. It communicates to your employees your clinic procedures, rules, expectations, goals, and philosophy. We have included a "Staff Policy" in the upcoming personnel section so you can see what this looks like.

Whatever the person has been told he/she has been hired to do, it is not enough to just provide a general job description while pointing to the front office, and asking her to handle it. This approach contains: no work context and background; no priorities; no clarification of responsibilities; no attention to the employee's authority and availability of resources; no training and supervision. Under these circumstances, it is not at all clear what the acupuncturist cares about, and, therefore, what the employee should care about. It is not even clear that the practitioner does care.

Not bothering to determine and convey one's practice goals, objectives, and expectations can be interpreted by staff to mean "not caring." However, more often than not, the practitioner cares, but is not comfortable with his/her role as administrator and supervisor. The practitioner prefers to simply be a treating practitioner. Most practitioners who enter a new position do not clearly understand their own roles as practice owners and are not "excellent managers." This has to be learned. It takes sometimes a year or two before people can completely understand their role.

To assist you in achieving successful objectives, we have included an outline of " Job Responsibilities," to help guide you and your personnel. *Volume II* expands this to include **specific** training and procedures for daily operations.

Train your staff in your objectives. Explain and show the job responsibilities to your assistants when you hire your staff. Stress your priorities.

The **key approaches to successful practice management** are "management by objectives," good communication, and team spirit.

---

15 Management Objectives:

1. Attract patients who will successfully benefit from your services, who will follow through with care, pay, get well, refer, and return if an old condition reappears or new conditions develop.

2. Give the quality of care which creates loyal and enthusiastic patients.

3. Exemplify safe practice.

4. Steadily increase new patients and services performed by: high visibility, communication, credibility, competency, desirability, and prosperity.

5. Orient and educate patients regarding benefits of your services and motivate them to refer.

6. Spread your message, using a marketing plan, advertising impact, and costs — to maximum effective value.

7. Foster employee "teamwork", built on incentives — producing excellent morale, patient care and services, referrals and new patients.

8. Maintain the proper proportion of expenses in relation to income production.

9. Set proper fees and implement them.

10. Have Clear financial policies and specific implementation of them.

11. Implement and expand effective telephone communication, over-the-counter scheduling, collections, and follow-up.

12. Maintain proper billing and insurance procedures.

13. Keep accurate and up-to-date records and patient management statistics.

14. Follow-through with collections from an accounts receivable aging analysis.

15. Keep your overall objectives of your practice plan and expansion in mind so that you and staff are up-to-date. Add or delete procedures, staff, trainings and classes, environmental designs, equipment, marketing, etc. as needed.

Keep these management objectives in mind. Post this list for staff and use this as a focus point for staff meetings.

Have your staff utilize the manual sets—particularly *Volume II, The Practice Building Front Office Procedure: Training and Reference Manual,* and *Volume III, Success with Insurance.* If you are fortunate enough to already have an excellent office manager, have him or her train your office assistants using the manuals as a reference training guide. Send your staff to practice management seminars which incorporate acupuncturists and their staffs into their programs. Medical collection seminars are invaluable for your office assistants. Acupuncture colleges offer business management classes for acupuncturists. As of this date, a number of the schools are using this manual as a business management textbook. Stay alert to future classes offered in the acupuncture colleges for the acupuncturists' front office managers.

Even after you have trained your staff and delegated well, you must spend time encouraging your personnel to assume more responsibility and to make valuable contributions to your practice. By giving them a sense of purpose ,direction, and a valuable role to fill in their lives, you can help them feel good about themselves; In turn, more is done with increased quality. You satisfy a very necessary human need to be valuable, needed, and wanted, which in turn inspires them to give that to others.

As your staff becomes fully informed and trained, they become "experts" in your practice. This gives staff a tremendous sense of accomplishment. You can further develop their sense of contribution and motivation through staff meetings. Keep the focus on teamwork, the objectives of good practice and clear priorities. Provide the climate for staff to input their ideas and suggestions for carrying out good patient care and other practice objectives. We have included a section on "Managing Staff through Staff Meetings, Supervision and Incentives" to assist you.

Good staff contribution and teamwork occurs because of job satisfaction and enrichment opportunities. These are developed by setting high standards and goals to meet, providing considerable autonomy and responsibility for doing the work, providing recognition and appreciation for achievement, and providing real opportunities for learning, participation, and further achievement.

The Hiring Process

1. **Your Intention**
    Make sure your intention is clear regarding what type of person you want to hire. Think about what that kind of person you want, what tone and reputation you want conveyed. What are you willing to pay for the one who represents you, will be the one who could make or break you, who could be your biggest promoter, your trouble shooter, and your right hand person who keeps your front office managed well and your patients enthusiastic? After you have considered these things, advertise who you want, and set up a time frame and place (your office) to interview and complete your hiring process. Set a deadline date. However, in doing so, don't settle for less than what you want. It will make a big difference in your practice. Ask for a resume in your ad. That way you can pre-screen the applicants before calling the top three.

2. **Job Description.**
    Review and know the specification and responsibilities for the job. The following positions are described in detail in **Volume II**:

    ■ Front desk position
    ■ Insurance or administrative assistant
    ■ Bookkeeper
    ■ Back office support
    ■ Office manager

    In many offices these jobs are combined.

3. **The Screening Process.**
    Screen your applicants before the interview. If they call, find out if they can work your hours, if they have the basic qualifications listed in your ad, and if they would like to work in a health care acupuncture practice. You may want to find out their minimum salary requirements to see if it is in your ball park for hiring an applicant.

4. **Job Application.** *
    Have them come in a half hour before your interview time to fill out the job application, which should be handwritten. "Handwriting" reveals what your applicant's written communications may look

like to you in the future. Is your applicant's handwriting neat, orderly, readable, clear, warm, accurate with details, thoughtful, or messy, disorganized, inaccurate, etc.?
(*Job Application Forms as well as an Interview Questionnaire are in the *Big Forms Packet*).

5.   **Interview Questionnaire.***
You may want to check off basic questions on the questionnaire for your first round of interview. On the callbacks or second interview, go through the two pages of in-depth interviewing. As an investment it will be a great savings later in time, energy, and money. Also have your applicant perform a typing test at the end of the interview to see if he/she is able to meet your requirements in speed, correct spelling and punctuation.

(* In the *Big Forms Packet*)

6.   **Checking References**
The practitioner can be easily victimized by employees whose credentials are not checked thoroughly, therefore contact former employers of your qualified applicant and hear what they have to say about him/her.

Reference checks provide answers to questions concerning the candidate's performance on previous jobs. They are also helpful in verifying information on the application blank and statements made during interviews, in checking on possible omissions of information, and in clarifying specific points. The three sources of reference are: 1) academic 2) personal 3) previous employers. With business references, checks made by telephone or in person are preferred to written responses. The writer of a reference letter may have little or no idea of your job requirements. Also, past employers are sometimes reluctant to write poor letters of reference. Be sure to ask former employers specific questions about the candidate's performance, and whether they would consider rehiring the person.

(A Past Employer Inquiry Form can be found in the *Big Forms Packet to* send.)

7. **Physical Examination**
    Arrange to have the applicant take a physical examination, if he/she is the final candidate for the job. This is usually the last step before hiring, as it is generally the most expensive one.

    The applicant's health and physical condition should be matched to the physical requirements of the job. You should have your final applicant examined by a physician before hiring. It's best that you are not that physician, for obvious reasons. The examination could reveal physical limitations which would limit job performance. It will also help you comply with your state's workers' compensation laws by providing a record of the employee's health at the time of hiring, and it could prevent compensation claims for any injury which occurred prior to his/her employment with you.

8. **Staff Policy and Salary Considerations.**
    In the first round of interviews, your "staff policy" will be useful in fielding questions from your applicants on your expectations and their benefits. When you have decided who you want to hire, you can present a copy of your "Staff Policy" in full and a salary proposal. In deciding upon your salary proposal take into consideration 1) the usual, customary, and reasonable rate for the position 2) the person's skills and experience, 3) trial time with a specific salary increase after passing the first review, 4) the person's opportunity to learn new skills and services, 5) opportunity for advancement of position and salary, 6) merit raises, 7) bonuses for meeting goals, 8) the yearly standard of living index and 9) your ability to pay. Any questions that need clarifying regarding your policy should be done at this time to avoid pitfalls in the future.

9. **Decision to Hire.**
    After completing the selection procedure, you are in a position to decide whether an applicant should be hired on a trial basis or rejected. Your final decision should be made only after a probationary period. This is usually between one and three months - depending on how long it takes to learn to perform the job acceptably. By that time, your employee should know your practice well enough to decide whether or not you are the best bet.

10. **Training**

Let your applicant know you 1) want them to take on increasing responsibility, 2) you can provide orientation for them to the best of your ability; and 3) provide them with a reference manual to assist them with the details. (**Volume II** is the "Training and Reference Manual" for the front office and its procedures).

11. **Final Hiring**

After the prearranged probationary period, reevaluate your employee's attitude and work, and see if that person best fits with your practice. This decision is vital, because you will invest a great deal of trust, time, money, and energy in this person.

12. **Time and wages.***

Have your employee keep track of his or her specific hours on a daily basis. These can be totaled on a weekly or bimonthly basis and the wages and deductions written in at the pay period. Your employee needs to fill out a W-4 Form so that you know what deductions to take out of his/her check. The wage deductions booklets can be obtained from your local federal and state tax offices.

At the end of the quarter, you will need to total his/her wages and deductions and then pay a portion of his/her taxes on the Employers Quarterly Returns.

Sometimes you may hire someone on a contractor basis to do specific work for you for a lump sum. In this case you would not withhold any taxes; the "contractor" would take care of his/her own taxes. However, any amount paid over $600 would need to be reported to the IRS on a 1099 Form.

*"How to Do Payroll" is included in **Volume II.**

*Interview, Hiring Questionnaires, and Wages Sheet in the Big Forms Packet are highly recommended.

Introduction

So many practices do not have a clear written staff policy, and, unfortunately, it has caused great confusion, misunderstandings, and underlying resentment on the part of the staff. Have a clear "Staff Policy". I've enclosed a copy of a model, originally written by Dr. David Singer,* which I have revised for acupuncturists. It has proved both successful and beneficial for all concerned.

Staff Policy

The acupuncturist's Front Office Assistant is an extension of the acupuncturist. We rely heavily upon you particularly to ensure that the patient flow in and out of the office, hour by hour and day by day, is smooth and uninterrupted. The main tool you have to accomplish this end is the appointment book which you must come to understand thoroughly. The acupuncturist's Front Office Assistant(s) "run" the office, permitting the acupuncturist to spend his/her hours helping the patients get well. Your duties include management of patient flow, insurance work, billing and posting of accounts, correspondence, shopping for supplies, errands, ordering supplies, cleaning the office, answering the phone, preparation and mailing of monthly statements, etc.

You will soon discover that a smoothly running and efficient office depends upon teamwork. To the greatest extent possible, each member of the team is assigned a role which complements our main goal—getting sick people well and once well, keeping them that way—and discretely encouraging them to refer other sick people that acupuncture can help. As you'll learn, acupuncture is effective in a much greater number of health problems than the public realizes.

I. Purpose

The purpose of the office is to help as many people as possible through care and patient education.

---

* Dr. David Singer, Chiropractor and President of Singer Consultants, states he has the largest consulting firm in the world for health practitioners, and has numerous acupuncture clients. For information, 1-800-221-0385.

II. Patient Relations and Communications

Patients' needs come first. Our patients come here because they are in ill health and pain. We need to convey an atmosphere of warmth, cheerfulness, friendliness and competence. Do everything you can to show them that you care about them. Remember their names as you would want everyone you know to remember yours. You must learn to leave your own problems at home. *Extraneous conversation, particularly among you who work with us, must be kept virtually nonexistent.*

Furthermore, most people are very sensitive about having their own problems and record exposed to public view. Accordingly give no patient the impression that his or her "case" might become the object of a conversation which can be overheard by others in the reception room or anywhere else.

Report patient's comments. Positive comments by patients about their improvement, the practitioner, any phase of their care, should be relayed back to the practitioner. Negative comments should also be relayed as they may signal an important misunderstanding of their care program. The acupuncturist wants to have an open relationship with the patients and to answer their questions.

Understand acupuncture. One of your jobs is to understand and become educated about acupuncture. All employees must read literature that will educate them in the benefits of acupuncture.

III. Salary

Employees hired on salary will initially be hired on a probationary basis. At the end of that time an evaluation will be done to determine the necessity of continuing with a raise. Salary and raises are based upon job performance and production (merit-office and individual). Each employee will have a job evaluation every six months.

The rate of pay for new employees hired on an hourly basis is as follows:

First three months   _____

Three months to six months   _____

Six month to a year   _____

Merit indicates increased proficiency allowing you to assume duties above and beyond your normal position, and a willingness to contribute to the growth of the practice, i.e. helping as many people as we possibly can.

Paychecks are received twice per month.

IV. Benefits

Holidays. The office will be closed New Year's Day, Memorial Day, July 4th, Labor Day, Thanksgiving Day and Christmas Day. If the office is closed on Monday, Wednesday and Friday, the hours of the following or previous day may be extended. Extra hours may be necessary before or after holidays to keep up with daily work. If a holiday involves the closing of the office on a weekday, the days off normally granted during the week must be cancelled. If the office is open on a legal holiday you will be paid double time. For part time employees if a holiday falls on a normal working day you will be paid the normal hourly wage for that day.

Vacations. Paid vacations will be granted as follows: After six months, one working week vacation (if part time: 3 days/week = 3 vacations days). No staff member will be allowed to be on vacation more than two working weeks at one time. Vacations or days off must be requested one month in advance. Vacations must be taken within 1 year of accrual or time will be lost.

Family Health Care for Full Time Employees. For staff working more than 15 hours per week (as a permanent job) your care is at no charge. Vitamins and supplies are 60% of retail fee. Insurance assignment plus $1.00 per office visit will be accepted for care for your immediate family, or if no insurance, the charge is one half of fee for services rendered. After leaving employment in this office for any reason, this policy holds for one month only.

Christmas Bonus.

	Full time	Part time
One to six months service	$40.00	$30.00
Six months to one year	$80.00	$40.00
One year to two years	$100.00	$55.00
Two to three or more years	$140.00	$60.00

V. Promptness

You are expected to be at the office no later than 30 minutes before patients are scheduled. This is very important time needed to review office goals and schedule for the day. If you are going to be late, call the office immediately. Excessive tardiness is grounds for termination of employment.

Office hours for treatment and consultation are as follows:

One hour is allowed for a lunch break.

VI. Absence

The absence of any one staff member from the office will place an added burden on the remaining staff members who will be expected to "cover" for whomever is absent. Absences must be restricted to emergencies such as serious illness. If a crisis arises you must notify the acupuncturist or Office Manager as to the need for your absence and solution to your absence. You are allowed six crisis (sick) days in one year. If absence exceeds six days in one year, your time will be reduced from vacation time. You will be paid for any crisis days left over after one year. Excessive absence will lead to termination of employment. This policy regarding crisis days applies to salaried personnel.

VII. Bonus System

Bonuses will be given when your weekly target(s) are met as reflected by statistics.

When you reach your target you will receive a bonus of 5% of your weekly salary.

Management bonuses are $5 and are set by the acupuncturist when applicable.

Team goals and bonuses will be applied and set at the office meeting once a week with the acupuncturist.

VIII. Agreements (personal)—Implicit vs. Explicit Agreements

No dating of a staff member or patient during initial care.

No discussing of patient health problems or personality outside office.

No conversation with co-workers about other co-workers.

No gossip.

No discussing of office statistics or interoffice personal communications outside staff.

No discussing your salary or bonuses with any other staff member or patient.

Look for and present solutions to your problems.

Only complain to someone who can do something about the problem.

Always know your goals and what is needed at any given time to reach them.

Answer phone by second ring.

There is no such thing as a "job" at this office.

New staff are to use a daily completion form after each shift for the first two weeks on the job.

Acknowledge all jobs not completed to either me or an Office Manager in a written form.

If there is inefficiency in any area or a lack of integrity, please communicate this to me or the Office Manager.

Eating at the front desk area is not permitted.

Unauthorized use of physical therapy machines is grounds for termination.

IX. Special Events

Occasionally our clinic may sponsor an outside public talk on such topics as nutrition or acupuncture and herbs. You will be given specific jobs to perform at the time of the talk. Attendance is expected and your support of the event is considered a function of your job. You will be paid your regular hourly wage during the time you attend the event. Also, for several days after the event, extra phoning will be required. Extra hours put in for phoning will be compensated.

X. Uniforms
(Optional, according to the acupuncturist's choice)

Office Assistants wear white smocks during their shifts. This acupuncturist will buy two smocks per year per employee.

Dresses or dress slacks only are appropriate office wear.

Remember: The way you dress has an effect on the way you feel and act. Think professional!

XII. Seminars

Staff members may be requested to attend seminars for their education. All expenses for such seminars will be covered, however, no payment will be made for hourly time spent.

We welcome you to our staff. We hope that you will view your function here as something more than a 9:00 to 5:00 job.

Managing and Developing Your Staff

The most effective way of managing staff is "management by objectives" and "management by walking around," (MBWA, a key concept in Peter's and Waterman's *In Search of Excellence*.) This is a combination of both formal and informal methods, which improves morale, productivity, and quality throughout your acupuncture practice.

Many practices take a haphazard approach to communications. They hold spontaneous meeting or discussion in response to a crisis, or challenge patient or internal problems. Essential staff which should be involved may be overlooked while the wrong staff members are invited to participate. To eliminate this communications problem in your practice, hold periodic meetings to review performance and progress towards overall practice goals.

For effective communications, encourage your staff to meet for ten minutes a day to review productivity, quality and other performance indicators. The larger the practice and staff, the more important it will be to coordinate and communicate through weekly meetings. Meetings keep staff informed and focused on the immediate goals.

Deliberate take the time for brief informal communication--MBWA, to browse and keep in touch with your front office staff, insurance billing staff, back office staff, or other vital members each day. Whether these jobs are combined into one person, keep informed about current affairs, without being overcontrolling. Observe how the font office person handles patents, listen to the way the phone is handled, how insurance collection is done. You'll learn a lot about how effective your family, staff, or employees are. Brief **one minute** encounters of encouragement, positive appreciation, listening to a victory they had, hearing a concern, lets your staff know you care. This brief time has a powerful impact on staff performance. It often is enough to keep their interest and enthusiasm alive in looking for new ways to improve their performance and your practice. They can give you valuable patient and office efficiency feedback so improvement can be made, and it gives you a chance to feel the steady pulse of your practice.

Whether your staff is family or non-family, staff need tlme to get to know you and other staff outside of their role. This is special time to get to appreciate one another as people. Often a practitioner will hold a yearly picnic with staff or occasionally take staff for lunch to get to know an employee on a personal level. It's the personal touch that makes a difference in your approach to employee communications. Ask about the employees personal goals, their children, any vacation plans. Build a more open and honest communication between you and your staff.

Make sure your staff has an opportunity to see you in action with patients when you do routine patient care, examination, a report of findings, etc. How can they promote you if they don't know how you are as a practitioner?!

We all thrive on open communication and care for one another. As long as this is present, you are "keeping"—caring for—your staff. Set a time on a regular basis to meet, and don't let other things crowd your meetings out of the schedule.

How to Produce Effective Staff Meetings

Staff Meetings are where the "creative juices flow", ideas are born, practice objectives are communicated, teamwork is initiated, grievances are cleared, and the door of communication is open just for and between staff in a confidential setting.

Guidelines for meetings:

1. Keep updated! Hold meetings. If you do not hold meetings at all or on a regular basis, problems slide and build up in a practice.

2. Set a consistent time each week at least to meet (for example,. Wednesdays 1-2 P.M.). In smaller practices, meetings may be much shorter.

3. Don't let other things crowd your meetings out of the schedule. Meetings are essential for communicating items that cannot be handled during busy practice hours.

4. Make sure everyone is aware of the date and time of the meeting and read your guidelines for the way business meetings are conducted.

5. One person should consistently keep notes on the meetings to 1) communicate this to the acupuncturist if he/she is not present, and 2) to use for future reference.

6. Another person should have the role of "keeping the meeting on track". This person runs through the agenda items, keeps conversation to the point, and reminds the group to stay within the time limit allotted for each topic.

7. Meetings generally should be focused by the acupuncturist, or a designated manager who keeps communication lines open between the acupuncturist and the staff.

8. Begin with an agenda in each meeting in order to keep the purpose and focus of the meeting on track. The focus should always relate back to and strengthen the objectives of the practice and the people in it.

9. Agree to stick to the agenda during the meeting unless there is a consensus that an item supersedes the agendas topics.

10. Have a "no interruption" policy during a meeting. Put the answering machine on. All other business can wait outside the room. Inside the room one person speaks at a time either at his/her turn if each person gets to speak on a topic. Wait until all have voiced their initial thoughts before listening to responses or reactions to the initial thoughts. Decide each meeting to let each person speak without interruption, unless getting off the agenda.

11. Listen carefully to each other. How can what the person is saying serve the practice? What does this one want or need? What do you want or need? Do you hear each other? Give yourselves enough time to address what is being said.

12. Make up the next agenda together for unfinished business — before the last meeting ends. Prioritize these items for future meeting dates.

13. Agenda topics may form throughout the week. If you have a number of items on the agenda, consider having more frequent meetings, particularly where pressing items need to be handled.

14. Consider new projects, direction, ways to serve the patients better and smoother functioning as a team.

15. Consider expansion and inclusion of new people in different ways — both in the office and in regards to outreach.

16. Keep the spirit of the team light. If your meetings are predominately issue oriented, deliberately schedule other types to balance out the energy in the office. Meet in different places — like over lunch, and out of the office. Set a date for staff picnics.

17. If you find you tend to avoid meetings, it may be time to communicate this and ask or help. It may be time to reorganize or let go of the way certain aspects of the office are. Don't hesitate to ask for a mediator or consultant to come in who can pull the energy of the office together.

18. Don't let anything stand in the way of enjoying working together! There is nothing that cannot be overcome with empathy, guidance, and humor.

Types of Meetings:

Morning:
- 1. Meditation - 3-5 minute circle of quiet energy.
- 2. Goal sharing.
- 3. Prioritizing goals.
- 4. Communication of carry over items from the day before.
- 5. Short review of the daily patient schedule.

Midday meeting - weekly, biweekly, one to one and a half hours:
- 1. Brainstorming.
- 2. Implementing a plan.
- 3. Office staff training/further education.
- 4. Reviewing old policies.
- 5. Rebuilding communication lines.
- 6. Personnel review.
- 7. Patient review.
- 8. Positive time management.
- 9. Financial review.
- 10. Setting new polices.
- 11. Ways of making the practice more efficient.
- 12. Patient education.
- 13. Planning an event, program, presentation.
- 14. Referral building.
- 15. Success stories.
- 16. Communication procedures.
- 17. Ways of expanding the practice.
- 18. Safe practice.
- 19. Reviewing what the "I"s all want; purpose review; and team building.

Employee Supervision and Review Process

(Evaluation of time use and performance, quality of service and merit raises.)

It is very important to make time on a regular basis to do the following:

1. Consideration and evaluation by the practitioner on a one to one basis.

2. Progress report.

3. Consideration of alternatives.

Review with your employee the following and build in rewards and incentives: In the first space write + or - or ? For strong, weak or areas where your awareness of their performance isn't clear. In the second space check areas which show that a merit, bonus, or raise is in order. Discuss areas which need improvement.

____ ____ Patient Rapport
____ ____ Promoting you and the practice
____ ____ Referral building and ability to make the practice grow
____ ____ Specific scheduling program to promote follow-through
____ ____ Telephone procedure, new patient recalls, backsliding proce
dure
____ ____ Handling financial arrangements
____ ____ Collection ability
____ ____ Patient follow-up procedure
____ ____ Handling front office flow, being a hub
____ ____ Handling interruptions well
____ ____ Knowledge of acupuncture benefits
____ ____ Orienting and educating patients, providing follow-through
pamphlets, answering patient questions
____ ____ Practices safe practice
____ ____ Problem Solving/ Troubleshooting
____ ____ Insurance billing and follow-through procedure
____ ____ Organizing prioritizing paperwork
____ ____ General material_____ Medical_____
____ ____ Knowledge of medical terminology
____ ____ Keeping accurate detailed records
____ ____ Keeping statistics and even analyzing them
____ ____ Filing
____ ____ Composing and editing letters

____ ____	Spelling
____ ____	Typing ____wpm accuracy ____
____ ____	Good with numbers
____ ____	Cleaning the office
____ ____	Dictation
____ ____	Back office work - paper
____ ____	Back office - patient care
____ ____	Giving direction
____ ____	Following direction
____ ____	Overview
____ ____	Detail work
____ ____	Speaks a foreign language (which one?)_____
____ ____	Health care training
____ ____	Public speaking ability for health care classes
____ ____	Offering in new ideas which are effective, efficient improve ments
____ ____	Ability to work well with you or other staff

To what extent has the employee demonstrated that he/she can or wants to accept grater autonomy and responsibility?

Review staff at regular intervals, such as at the end of a probationary or trial-hire, at three months, six months, and yearly intervals.

Refer to your staff policy when looking at staff performance and their ability to met your standards. This is a written form of expectations to which your staff can hold themselves accountable. Review your staff's performance in the light of your staff policy as well. Fulfill your promises and commitments written in your staff policy. This must be a win-win situation for staff to continue to be with you year after year. Staff appreciate your willingness to give them review, and your willingness to offer merit, incentives, job enrichment, job satisfaction warranted raises, appreciation for a job well done, and the opportunities to profit share or benefit as the practice grows.

Staff Encouragement, Motivation, and Incentives

Team spirit is the key. Communicate the mission of your practice and how each person is part of that mission. Give them opportunities to communicate how they can fulfill it.

1. Invite your personnel to think of the job in terms of accomplishment rather than merely activity.

2. Solicit the employee's ideas on ways to increase the contribution he/she can make to the practice by means of his/her activities.

3. Encourage each employee to plan out those aspects of his/her job which are not matters of routine. Have the employee communicate how he/she will accomplish the task (i.e. P.R. program, referral generation, etc.) and what measures of achievement he/she will use to assess his/her work. Be willing to give a bonus for scheduling those "new" patients because of excellent front office promotion work.

4. Encourage cost saving or efficiency steps.

5. Reward accomplishment, not merely activity. Give compliments for a job well done. Be free with praise and honest compliments. Don't overdo it, but don't under do it either.

6. Communicate high expectations. Make performance an organization ethic. Talk about it, specify it, require it, and reward it. Try in every way possible to reward employees for independent problem solving and acceptance of responsibility. By action and interactions, create and maintain an atmosphere which permits honest mistakes. Be quick to reward and slow to punish.

7. When you hold a review conference with the individual employee, give the employee a chance to clarify his/her thinking. This can help you see how to communicate your objectives more clearly to your employee and to understand what you both may have assumed he/she understood but didn't. Use you review session to spark enthusiasm to clearer or new objectives.

8. Give your employees ample opportunity to see how much they can grow and see a future with your practice. Having written staff policy benefits provides security Try building in a profit sharing plan. Remember: One of your biggest worthwhile investments is in the keeping of good staff.

Staff Incentive, Benefits, and Rewards

1. Bonus of $25 for referral of a new patient who continues at least four times.

2. Bonus of 1% of monthly payments to each practitioner over $6,000 to be split between the office staff.

3. After the first ___(six months, 1 year) 1 week paid vacation.

4. After the second year, 2 weeks paid vacation.

5. Acupuncture benefits free of charge for staff's immediate family and staff if already uninsured. All deductibles and co-payment waived if under current insurance.

6. Supplements at 60% off retail (or at cost) for self and immediate family.

7. 7 days paid sick leave during the first year.

8. 10 days paid sick leave after the first year.

9. Uniform allowance in place of equal time of labor (i.e. specific amount not subject to take out of pay taxes each month.) See tax accountant for the legal limit per year.

10. Christmas bonus.

Recap

In the section on staff, we have discussed the value of hiring and keeping good staff, and the importance of having staff who are 1) oriented to your objectives, and 2) able to show a high level of patient rapport, business skill, and team spirit.

We have considered both the benefits of delegating and the pitfalls of poor delegation. We've looked at the solution then of hiring appropriate staff, reevaluating effective staffing, communicating what you want for your practice to your employees, what kind of results you want to see, and providing 1) training, 2) supervision, 3) motivation, 4) monitoring, and 5) ample appreciation. The following questionnaire will help you focus your actions.

Hiring, Delegating, Staff Decisions Questionnaire

1. What hiring decisions can you make which will free you to practice with less stress, greater patient service, and greater profitability?_____
   _____

2. What personnel changes must you make to allow your practice to grow?_____
   _____

3. What delegating decisions will you make to reduce your stress?
   _____
   _____

4. What delegating decisions will you make to increase better patient   service?
   _____
   _____
   _____

5. What delegating decisions will you make to increase your profitability?
   _____
   _____

6. If you have to manage one area that prevents your practice from better service and profit -- avoiding conflict/needing to please, need to control, need to hire weaker staff than self, what will you do about it? _____
   _____

7. How will you get feedback from your staff, monitor your practice, and ensure staff carries out your objectives?_____
   _____

8. What philosophy objectives, and incentives can you provide fo employees to give better care, increase your practice growth, and financial collections?_____
   _____

9. What other decisions must you make to increse team spirit?_____
   _____

Controlling and Delegating Aptitude / Next Steps Questionnaire

1. Please indicate your skill and substanial positive experience level in each of the following
   areas: strong = + questionable = ? poor = -

2. Then indicate your interest level in each of the following areas.
   like = + questionable = ? avoid = -

3. Indicate who will handle the area, when, costs, level of skill needed-- high, moderate, low

Skill Level	Interest Level	Area/Field	First Action Step -- Who will handle, # days/hrs.per month, Hourly / Mo. Costs
_____	_____	1. Acupuncture - related Therapy	_____
_____	_____	2. Planning	_____
_____	_____	3. Networking	_____
_____	_____	4. Referral Building	_____
_____	_____	5. Budgeting	_____
_____	_____	6. Accounting, expenses	_____
_____	_____	7. Outside Public Relations/Adverstising	_____
_____	_____	8. Marketing	_____
_____	_____	9. Design/Aesthetics	_____
_____	_____	10. Administration -- Supervision/Delegat- ing, Staff Meetings	_____
_____	_____	11. Organizing	_____
_____	_____	12. Front Office Manage- ment & Control	_____
_____	_____	13. Telephone procedure	_____
_____	_____	14. Patient Set Up	_____
_____	_____	15. Patient Reception, Intake & Scheduling	_____
_____	_____	16. Patient Follow-up	_____
_____	_____	17. Paperwork Processing	_____
_____	_____	18. Typing/Filing	_____
_____	_____	19. In house Collections	_____
_____	_____	20. Patient Billing	_____
_____	_____	21. Patient Insurance	_____
_____	_____	22. Patient Orientation and Education	_____
_____	_____	23. Teaching	_____
_____	_____	24. Investing	_____
_____	_____	25. Research	_____
_____	_____	26. Legal Aspects	_____
_____	_____	27. Taxes	_____
_____	_____	28. Business overiew	_____

Poor or questionable interest in the above areas could indicate need for interest/skills
development and/or careful delegation.

PRACTICE MANAGEMENT PERSPECTIVE

Management Control

Practice management includes a number of areas. Income and outflow and the right proportion of income to expenses are major aspects.

You will avoid expense, time waste, and energy by making sure you have hired the right professional assistance. These employees prove effective in their attitude, their ability to build agreement, in their care for people, and are accurate and efficient in handling the daily affairs of your practice. Take the time to hire the right people.

Hire staff, but don't hire a full time staff person from start unless you have a built in practice you have just taken over. Increase staff hours as your practice permits. Make sure staff job descriptions and goals are written and clear implemented. Schedule a weekly staff meeting. Use your calendar to prioritize and set deadlines to make sure things are done.

A practitioner must setup management control to insure that the right things are done on a day to day basis. (Note the control forms in the *Big Forms Packet*).

Look at your procedures. Are they efficient and effective? Look at your fees and how they are implemented. Look at your financial policy and how it is carried out. Look at how you are scheduling your patients, as well as the way fees are collected. Do you have proper billing procedures and collections from accounts receivable aging analysis? What could be upgraded?

Look to see: Are patients referring other patients? Are you using marketing tools to educate patients about acupuncture and you? Is your assistant encouraging new patients or is he or she overworked? Are you, as a practitioner, keeping current on new data to treat patients? Are you expanding your range of services to your patients? Is your rapport with your patients all that it could be? What can you do to be more effective as a treating practitioner that would allow more patients to get well? All these affect your practice profitability, as well as your reputation and your practice success.

Use the "Creating Successful Practice Section" to **focus your efforts.**
Use pages 37-40; 76; 87, 113-118; 326-327 to **set your goals.**
Use "Pitfalls to Avoid for Successful Practice" to help **monitor your practice.**

What to Monitor

- QUALITY AND SUCCESS of professional patient services and treatment.

- Quality control of PATIENT SERVICE by staff

- EFFECTIVENESS of office procedures

- FEEDBACK from patients and staff *

- EFFICIENCY AND TIMING
  In-office patient flow. Staff's organizational ability with record-handling, paperwork, and the phone. Appointment booking. Patient education and orientation. Bookkeeping and billing system. Insurance processing system. Advertising methods and referral building procedures.

- VOLUME AND TURNOVER
  Appointment management control *
  Patient volume. Missed cancelled, and rescheduled appointments. Patient reactivation. Rescheduling follow-through. Reason for rise and drops.

- CASH FLOW *
  Ability to pay expenses. Steady cash in the bank. Accounts receivable outstanding and the length they are non-liquid. Type of income and percentages--cash up front, to general insurance, to long term litigation, to trades, to unstable cash (sliding scale); percentage of collections--ratio to what's outstanding: Follow-up procedures.

- FINANCIAL BALANCE
  Ability to get credit, borrow, and pay back. Ability to promote growth, expand, or level off. Tax planning advantages. Ratio of assets to financial liabilities.* Ratio of ACTUAL income to expenses. * Consider net **after** taxes!

- RESPONSE to type of marketing thrust, specialty emphasis *
  Type of patient referrals. Percentage of acute care patients to chronic and maintenance care. Ratio of new patients to turnover.

* To be found in the _Big Forms Packet_

In **Volume I** and particularly in the *Big Forms Packet* are forms to build practice management control into your practice. Your staff simply records totals from the "daily accounting and appointment sheets." An exceptional office manager and a good accountant can help you manage the adjustments to be made in your practice.

What if You Don't Monitor Your Practice?

1.   How much is your marginal staff member costing your practice in recalls, missed appointments, patient dissatisfaction, underdeveloped patient relationships, and return visit loyalty?

2.   How many more patients would you have this month if you had actively promoted referrals from your current patients, and thoroughly followed up on each interested patient lead?

3.   How much of an increase in patient visits and patient base could your practice realize if you had a strategic plan to develop a maintenance care program?

4.   How many new patients and/or loyal patients could you develop with a strategic plan to follow up on every patient?

5.   How much would your practice benefit from a plan that included training your staff in internal marketing?

6.   How much would your patient volume increase if you could motivate your front desk assistant to prevent backsliding for five patients who <u>need</u> your services, per week?

Doing recalls, rescheduling appointments, following through on patient needs, promoting referrals from current patients, following-up interested patient leads, maintenance care programs, internal marketing,etc. are not just good ideas. They all serve the patients needs and create valuable dollars every day, and are necessary to run and expand the practice. They also bring a profit back to the practitioner for a job well done.

How Patient Care Affects Practice Growth

Dr. Fernandez, PMA Consultant, cites five areas which either increase or decrease practice growth and income:

Total Patient Volume

Reason for Increase of Volume:

Tender loving care, keeping present patients coming for their benefit, motivating commitment and consistency in tending to a treatment program. Doing recalls, newsletters, a written reevaluation report.

Reason for Decrease:

Improper or lack of communication with patients, rushing patient, too high fees, lack of goals, not expressing results of acupuncture. No recall system. Short changing patient by not giving the time and consideration he/she deserves.

Total New Patients.

Reason for increase of new patients:

Excellent, thorough, well-planned consultation, examination, verbal and written Report of Findings, aliveness, telling about results in similar situations, Tender loving care, motivating commitment and clear patient communication, and good solid referral communication from the acupuncturist and staff.

Reason for decrease of new patients:

Poor consultation/exam, no written report, quick verbal report, no referral concept, no touch and tell procedures, no encouragement or mention of results.

**Total Weekly
Income**

Reason for increase of volume:

A rise in total patient volume and new patients, expanding your services, such as counseling and physiotherapy, nutrition, and a planned collection system, improving clear financial agreements and follow through.

Reason for decline of income:

Decline in total patient volume and new patients, poor collection procedure, feeling of not having enough, of not being able to ask your patient for results or income.

**Total
Patient Dropout**

Reason for increase in patient dropout:

Poor service to patient, unimpressive consultation, exam and reports, poor communication about procedures and results, poor appointment system, office not on time, no patient control, no recall system, no reexaminations, just being a technician.

Reason for decrease in dropout:

Good recall system, educating, retraining patient into excellent habits, reexamining, eliminating long waits.

**Total
Patient Recall**

Reason for increase:

By telephone, by reminder card, office responds to missed or cancelled appointments immediately.

Reason for decrease:
No recall system. No patient control.

Patient Survey
Getting Feedback From Your Patients

Many practitioners think that because they don't hear any complaints or their front office assistant doesn't hear any complaints, that everything is fine with the practice--especially when the appointment book appears full. However, don't be fooled. The only way to know how your patients feel about you and your practice is to ask. You may be surprised! The following questionnaire can be put simply in the reception room for optional answering. However, the best results in getting feedback occur when patients are gracefully asked to fill out the questionnaire. Make it policy to ask the patient who has had at least one reevaluation visit. It's the best feedback you can get!

This questionnaire can tell you :

1. What patient conditions you tend to attract most and the patient's feeling on the level of successful results.

2. How your patients currently feel about their care in your practice and your practice in general. This can serve you to find out if you are currently on track, or else help you to add the touches and elements which would improve your practice feeling, expertise, image, and reputation.

3. What your patients want most in a practitioner and his/her practice.

4. Why they do or don't refer.

5. How much your patients know about your background and training.

6. Why your practice is growing or slowing down it's growth.

*If your rating is good or very good, several positive outcomes are **more likely** to occur:*

1. Patients will be reminded to refer to you.

2. It will reinforce their positive feelings about you.

3. It can provide you with testimonial material which you can use in a testimonial book or articles you write.

4. It can tell you what patients like best about you and your office and what is unique about your practice. This is difficult to be objective about, so it is helpful to hear it from patients. This is vital feedback which tells you what to emphasize in any marketing and advertising you do.

If you receive average to poor ratings in any area:

1. It can tell you more about what your patients are looking for most in a health care provider.

2. How you or your practice can improve.

3. Why they may hesitate to refer.

4. It can tell you that you provide what they expect, but not necessarily what makes them feel enthusiastic about a practitioner.

* We Appreciate Feedback From Our Patients *
Please Fill This Out

Because we want to give you the very best of service, you can help us to serve you better by giving us feedback. We know that listening to our patients is the best way we can keep our standards high and give you the best.

1. What kind of condition did you come to us for: _____

2. What is your opinion on the following:

	very good	good	average	poor	don't know
Preparation and Considerateness of You When Treating					
Recommendations and Instructions					
Schedule towards Your Health Care Goals					
Supplemental Education or Literature					
Progress Evaluation					
Successful Results with Care					
Appointment System (promptness and availability)					
Reception Room (comfort and convenience)					
Professional Assistants (courtesy and competence)					
Special Services and Equipment					
Parking and Location					
Office Appearance					

3. Will you recommend us to your friends and family? ___ Yes ___ No

4. What are the goodies or "extras" which make our office and your acupuncturist special? _____
_____

May we quote you? ___ Yes ___ No _____ (Your name, unless you prefer to be anonymous)

5. How did you happen to come to our acupuncturist? ___ Friend's recommendation ___ Know him/her personally ___ Physician referral ___ Read article by or about him/her ___ Ad ___ Heard him/her speak ___ Telephone book ___ Other

6. What do you like best about your acupuncturist? _____

7. What could be improved about your acupuncturist? _____

8. What's most important to you when you come to a health care provider? _____

9. How many years of training do you think are required for acupuncture licensure? ___ for oriental medicine? _____

10. Your acupuncturist adds to his services by undertaking post-graduates seminars to keep up to date in practice. How many hours do you imagine your acupuncturist spends each year on keeping up to date? _____

11. How much investment would you guess your acupuncturist has in office equipment and professional facilities? _____

12. Any other comments you would like to add? _____

Thank you for taking the time to help us to serve you better!

Pitfalls to Avoid for Successful Practice

Often when something is off, we can't see it from the standpoint of what creates successful practice. It can be seen from looking at the omissions. If you have problems in your practice or want to avoid them, one of the first things to do is to discover what the problem is or potential problems are so you build in your solutions!

This list is extensive and quite complete. It is not intended to be used to beat yourself up for what you haven't done. After all, we aren't here to be perfectionists, but to offer the best we can with what we have to work. Remember: With all that you find you want to do differently, there is much that is right and special about your practice. Focus on what's right and uniquely you -- and add to your practice, one step or procedure at a time. We recommend that you don't throw away anything in your practice that works just because of seeing new ways of doing things.

The check mark system can help you overview and then get specific; so make notes for any first steps you will take to add to your practice. Almost anything can be uplifted by positive change and openness to feedback!

Correctable Structural and Functional Problems: Practice balance of type of patients, volume, turnover, cash flow, and energy flow

    Predominately acute care practice, niche market, high turnover practice, no referral building or effective advertising, with high or low fees, good or poor location

    Chronic care practice, low turnover, but predominately Medicare or low socioeconomic income area

❑ Drop in practice, no appointment necessary

❑ Crisis practice, high emergencies, erratic schedule, focus on house calls
    (loss time in unpaid travel)

❑ Sliding fee practices, mostly low end income

❑ Assignment of insurance payment only practices, with or without waiving deductible

❑ No insurance system practice

❑ No workers' compensation practice development, unless strong niche market for your specialty)

- ❑ Quality practice, high volume, overstuffed waiting rooms, no second or more treating practitioner
- ❑ Quality practice, low volume, high rent and lease payments, no networking or referral exchange or referral building, no niche market or advertising to such
- ❑ Quantity practice, minimal service or amenities, overstuffed waiting rooms, no second or more treating practitioners, patient switching, poor follow-through

Reputation Pitfalls
- ❑ No reputation, unknown
- ❑ Inconsistent
- ❑ Poor reputation
- ❑ Scary reputation of malpractice or negligence
- ❑ Womanizer
- ❑ Outdated
- ❑ Negative -- bossy, know-it all attitude, too preachy, inflexible, high-pressure, too rushed
- ❑ Too lax, too unspecific
- ❑ Too eccentric
- ❑ Regimented practice

Practitioner's Image
- ❑ Unspecific identity, difficult for others to describe you
- ❑ No niche market
- ❑ No specialties
- ❑ Nonprofessional dresser
- ❑ Nonprofessional attitude or mannerisms
- ❑ Outdated
- ❑ Inconsistent with appearance of self, office, location, equipment, and advertising
- ❑ Not knowing how to communicate to others about your practice
- ❑ No brochures, no advertising about you
- ❑ Office and location are functional only and do not convey your interests, expertise, your love of people
- ❑ Labeled as poor man's doctor, rich-man's doctor; rules out the middle class

PRACTICE ADMINISTRATIVE AND MANAGEMENT PROBLEMS

Practice Planning Approach
- ❏ Attempting too much at once/ not handling duties in chunks or clusters of time/ fractionalizing time/ Unrealistic time estimates
- ❏ No practice plan
- ❏ No deadlines/ day dreaming
- ❏ Fire fighting/ Crisis management
- ❏ Leaving tasks unfinished inappropriately
- ❏ Wasting time by shifting priorities
- ❏ No Objectives, priorities, or daily plan

Financial Planning and Management
- ❏ No, poor, erratic financial planning
- ❏ Not borrowing enough when beginning practice
- ❏ Income out of balance with outflow without controlled planning
- ❏ No phase-in practice planning
- ❏ No or poor planning for economic stabilization
- ❏ No or poor planning to handle influx of growth
- ❏ No or poor planning for reducing economic stress of growth
- ❏ No or poor planning of expenses and budgeting
- ❏ Not adjusting unrealistic income expectations until far into debt
- ❏ No financial management controls for accounts receivable or accounts payable -- profit and loss statements, (control forms in Forms Packet)
- ❏ Not calling in financial advisor for help
- ❏ No CPA, bookkeeper, lawyer on your team
- ❏ Not seeing income as "actual after tax income", instead of gross, so overspending
- ❏ Not putting funds aside for taxes -- payroll, general
- ❏ Not getting or cutting out insurance payments, including malpractice
- ❏ Funds tied up back end payments and in lengthy litigation cases,
- ❏ High accounts receivables, low cash, not enough cash to pay bills (Accounts receivables should be about 3 times gross plus 10%)
- ❏ Low accounts receivable, low cash, not enough cash to pay the bills
- ❏ Low volume practice, not enough cash to pay the bills
- ❏ High turnover, little new patients, not enough to pay the bills
- ❏ Income imbalance from patient type, volume, turnover, and energy flow
- ❏ Using procedures, equipment, buildings, office space that increase overhead excessively

- ❏ Leasing expensive little used equipment
- ❏ Leasing inexpensive equipment instead of buying it.
- ❏ Leasing unnecessary equipment,
- ❏ Overstocking anything
- ❏ Getting more new stock, using new, instead of moving old stock
- ❏ Type of advertising expenses don't justify new patient counts

Outreach Planning and Management
- ❏ Not looking at one's reputation and finding ways to build it
- ❏ Not clarifying and identifying one's image
- ❏ Not defining a specialty and marketing to a niche
- ❏ No marketing plan
- ❏ No or poorly planned and carried out in-house referral building procedure
- ❏ No or poor advertising
- ❏ No consultation or marketing advice from a professional

Procedure and Policy Planning, Set Up, and Implementation
- ❏ No or very little clear guidance or direction in setting up effective procedure and policy
- ❏ No written policy, procedure guide (Volume I, II and forms packets are now available)
- ❏ Right attitude in staff carrying out poor policy
- ❏ Poor attitude in staff carrying out the right policies
- ❏ No monitoring, correction in attitude, policy, procedure, or priorities

Organizing Practice or Daily Routine
- ❏ Confused responsibilities and authority
- ❏ Duplication of effort
- ❏ Personal Disorganization/ Stacked Desk
- ❏ Multiple authority figures with whom to coordinate in multiple practitioner office

Staffing
- ❏ Personnel with problems
- ❏ Understaffed / Overstaffed
- ❏ Untrained/ Inadequate staff
- ❏ Competition with or between staff
- ❏ Unappreciated staff
- ❏ Surrounding self with weak people instead of stronger people

Directing Your Practice
- ❏ Not coping with change
- ❏ Not managing conflict
- ❏ No coordination / No teamwork
- ❏ Lack of motivation
- ❏ Ineffective delegation
- ❏ Involved in routine details; poor supervision of practice
- ❏ Doing it all yourself
- ❏ Moving too fast; losing rapport;
- ❏ Missing specific details that spell good patient care and good practice management
- ❏ Not giving patients any direction(s) for better care

Controlling Your Practice
- ❏ Can't let go to let others do tasks better or different than you would.
- ❏ Wasting time by telephone/ Visitors
- ❏ Wasting time by incomplete information
- ❏ No standards or progress reports for the practice
- ❏ No review of management controls
- ❏ Overcontrol
- ❏ Mistakes/ Ineffective performance
- ❏ Overlooking poor performance of staff
- ❏ Inability to say "no" to patients or staff, "too nice", can't fire staff
- ❏ Not comfortable making recommendations to patients
- ❏ Patients take control with blabbing, inability to crystallize the need and act
- ❏ Not wanting to deal with hiring, training, or keeping your staff

Communicating
- ❏ Off-purpose with patients, staff, way of referral building or advertising, Lack of Professionalism , Lack of confidentiality
- ❏ Wasting time in Meetings
- ❏ Gabbing unproductively with patients about self, not the patient
- ❏ Under --, Over --, and Unclear Communicating, (Talk too much, not enough, not clear enough, with patients and/or staff)

- ❏ Don't listen enough
- ❏ Failure to Listen
- ❏ Wasting time by Socializing

Decision Making

- ❏ Snap decisions with patients, staff, accountant, others
- ❏ Indecision/ Procrastinating with patient treatment care and treatment planning, with practice procedure and policy changes, with staffing, with financial decisions, referral building and marketing
- ❏ Wanting all the facts
- ❏ Red tape waiting for others to move first before you can decide
- ❏ Decision by superiors or preferred group, inhibiting your decision and action
- ❏ Unpopular decisions defeating faith, acceptance, and action by others

PHYSIOGRAPHICAL PROBLEMS

Location Pitfalls

- ❏ City, county, state or country you reside in is too limiting legally or in attitude for your practice desires and potential
- ❏ Overlooking an area or other areas which would be better for your specialty
- ❏ Acupuncture plus specialty or niche doesn't fit for socioeconomic area
- ❏ Inaccessible or inconvenient area for your niche market
- ❏ Undesirable or unpreferred area for your specialty
- ❏ No parking or difficult parking,
- ❏ Second floor, stairs, no elevator
- ❏ Can't read your sign
- ❏ Poor growth potential,
- ❏ Declining neighborhood
- ❏ Wrong zone to practice
- ❏ Area has a history of unsuccessful practices
- ❏ Oversaturated area with practitioners like you
- ❏ Not enough population base to support your practice

Office Space

- ❏ Rent disproportionate to needs and ability to afford
- ❏ Functional office in high status neighborhood
- ❏ Overdone office in low status neighborhood
- ❏ Poor layout, can't expand or adapt well
- ❏ Too small, too unadaptable presently
- ❏ Problem with future addition
- ❏ Economically difficult rent or lease arrangement
- ❏ Can't sublet, lease-option, buy

❑ Space too run-down, poor heating/ cooling/ water/ toilet system
❑ Entire building maintenance and management problems

SUBJECTIVE PRACTICE PROBLEMS

Office Image Pitfalls
❑ Staff or practitioner non-professionally dressed
❑ Functional only, unaesthetic, office appearance
❑ Empty feeling facilities
❑ Dead appearance, no plants, color, light, or interesting magazines
❑ Disorganized office image
❑ Office too crowded or too empty
❑ Detained patients sitting in "waiting room"
❑ Outdated or worn appearance
❑ Rushed office feel
❑ Unclean or distasteful office image
❑ Excessively overdone facilities
❑ Cramped facilities
❑ No regular office upkeep, paint, carpet
❑ Lack of freshness, musty, stuffy, moxa, stale smelling
❑ Freezing, boiling, uncomfortable feeling
❑ Front office doesn't show both practitioner's specialty or true character

PROCEDURAL AND POLICY PROBLEMS

Telephone Procedures
❑ No yellow page listing in the phone book; people don't know your number
❑ No answering machine or voice mail
❑ Answering machine turned off
❑ Poorly communicated answering machine tape messages
❑ No rotating emergency on call procedure with other practitioners
❑ No call forwarding system
❑ Untimely call backs, or erratic call backs
❑ Phone conversations taking precedent over patients standing and waiting at the front desk.
❑ No protocol for handling calls in a multiple practitioner office
❑ No standard for dialogue procedures
❑ No training for handling new patient calls, handling problem patients, insurance company calls
❑ Assistant doesn't know how to promote you or your practice to new patients

- ❏ Assistant doesn't know how to prepare a new patient before arriving in your office.
- ❏ Assistant doesn't know how to answer qestions about you or your practice over the phone.
- ❏ Not knowing how to prevent backsliding when phone rescheduling
- ❏ Not doing phone follow-up of collections
- ❏ Not checking-up on the new patient, or no call to reactivate maintenance checks on former patients.

Front Office Patient Intake and Outgo Procedure
- ❏ Impersonal and indifferent attitude of staff; Patients treated like a number
- ❏ Long waits for practitioner and at the front desk outgoing
- ❏ No amenities, herb tea, water, magazines while waiting
- ❏ Patients rushed in and out
- ❏ No preparation or dialogue about treatment or literature given about the practice
- ❏ No written or verbal explanation of policy, procedures, insurance handling
- ❏ Information on "Patient Introduction and History" missed, incomplete, unchecked, no "Patient Report " filled in,
- ❏ No consent or authorization forms signed or checked.
- ❏ Files lost, misplaced, unprepared for the practitioner
- ❏ No patient education forms given
- ❏ No reinforcement of benefits from care
- ❏ No requests for referral asked or courtesy consultation cards promoted
- ❏ No explanation of equipment and audiovisual aids for patient benefit.
- ❏ Front office person doesn't get paperwork prepared for practitioner(s) in a timely way
- ❏ Too busy attitude.
- ❏ Paperwork, phone, taking precedent over the patient in the office
- ❏ Confusion, misunderstandings

Patient Care Procedures
- ❏ (See communication)
- ❏ Little or no compassion, understanding, hope, assurance, reinforcement given to patients
- ❏ Little or no explanation of benefits of procedure and care
- ❏ Little or no touch and tell procedures
- ❏ No patient program or preplanned visits
- ❏ No report of findings
- ❏ Oral and written report of findings, schedule, and recommendations not prepared and ready for second visit

- Little or no recommendations for home care, classes, treatment enhancement, products which support care
- Not wanting to take time to recommend; or fear of recommending
- No direction sheets or explanation of do's and don'ts for health care
- No reevaluation visits
- Limit or don't raise level of competency in weak areas of treatment
- Not scheduling intensified treatment, spreading visits out too far
- Releasing patients prematurely
- Keeping patients coming too much
- Forgetting to give the patient their next visit time
- Demanding or fear of demanding an unrealistic schedule of care
- Not getting a second opinion when unclear
- No follow-up reactivation or maintenance program
- Appointments rushed and too short for proper care
- Appointments too lengthy for busy people
- Giving patient tattered gowns, no gowns
- Too much additional therapy or nutrition
- Lack of professionalism

Unsafe Practice Procedure
- No explanation of benefits and hazards of acupuncture or rationale for treatment
- No or poor patient feedback mechanisms built into your practice
- No consent or authorization forms signed for treatment or check system for this
- Practicing beyond one's scope; treating by unacceptable, illegal or unauthorized procedures
- Myopic. Not keeping up to date with current information in the medical field
- Thinking your way of treating is the only way
- Letting patients dictate treatment
- Assistant not present in compromising circumstances
- Unreturned phone calls of critical nature
- Dismissing patient without a needed referral; abandonment
- Poor history and other forms which don't assist you to prevent or solve problems
- No recording of diagnosis and treatment rationale
- Poor recording procedure by patient and practitioner
- Don't refer judiciously
- Use untrained assistants

- ❏ Office staff advises without your consent
- ❏ No office staff policy to alert you when there are troublesome patients.
- ❏ Poor care from rushing
- ❏ Not bringing overbooking in check by hiring another practitioner, or raising fees to compensate by raising quality and giving extra time
- ❏ Not consulting with concurrent practitioner
- ❏ Not getting a second opinion when unclear
- ❏ Poor needle technique and poorly timed needle removal
- ❏ Poor sterilization technique
- ❏ Negligence and patient injury
- ❏ Dangerous waste disposal procedure
- ❏ Reacting to patient threats of suit without counsel
- ❏ Letting malpractice insurance go

Scheduling Procedures
- ❏ Peak patient times not considered when setting up days and hours
- ❏ Schedule is exhausting, long hours, too spread out, no days off
- ❏ Schedule is too cramped, days too short, not regular enough for patient care
- ❏ Not scheduling patients or paperwork in clusters
- ❏ Not having a time allotment system for patient type -- new ,established, injury
- ❏ Overbooking patients
- ❏ Off schedule
- ❏ Always late
- ❏ Keeping patients waiting more than 15 minutes
- ❏ Not scheduling a patient, patient drops out prematurely
- ❏ Assistant lets patients leave without scheduling or checking with practitioner about next visit or series.
- ❏ No recommendations for scheduling
- ❏ No multiple appointment schedule system with patients
- ❏ Missing call backs
- ❏ No follow-up system or care after cancellations
- ❏ No backsliding prevention scheduling
- ❏ No patient reminder system or maintenance care check appointed
- ❏ Not scheduling regular short office meetings

Financial Policy and Procedures
- ❏ Cash only policy
- ❏ No mastercard/ visa setup

- ❑ Demanding large up-front cash payments
- ❑ No payment plans
- ❑ No , over , under, unclearly -- communicated financial policies
- ❑ No discussion or explanation of fees
- ❑ "Take it or leave it" communication of fees
- ❑ No written financial agreements
- ❑ No assignment of benefits, 60 day courtesy
- ❑ Fees too high
- ❑ First visit too high, turns new patients away
- ❑ Inconsistent , always changeable financial policy
- ❑ Unmonitored financial policy implementation
- ❑ No trades
- ❑ Too many free services
- ❑ Practitioner unrecorded procedures

Recording and Billing Procedures
- ❑ Inconsistent and irregular financial recording
- ❑ Assistant unbilled or misbilled procedures
- ❑ Untimed mailing-out of patient and insurance billing
- ❑ Incomplete patient and insurance billings
- ❑ No or poor accounting control
- ❑ No monthly statistics , breakdown, and analysis of accounts receivable

Collection Procedures
- ❑ Afraid to ask for payment
- ❑ No collection training and good dialogue practice
- ❑ Not asking for payment at the time of service
- ❑ Inconsistent collection procedures
- ❑ Lost , misfiled, misplaced ledgers
- ❑ Unbalanced accounts
- ❑ No aging of accounts
- ❑ Poor or no follow-up procedures
- ❑ No collection statistics

Patient Insurance and Reporting Procedure
- ❑ No "Verification of Insurance Forms" given patient or checked
- ❑ No authorization for workers' compensation cleared
- ❑ No assignment of benefits, office insurance agreement, or liens signed
- ❑ Insurance form and bills lost, incomplete, misbilled, not followed up
- ❑ Patient doesn't know the status of their insurance payment and account with the office.

- ❑ Patient confused about insurance handling. No patient written or verbal explanation to assist.
- ❑ Late bills or no reports to insurance companies
- ❑ Poor history and treatment care record forms
- ❑ Poor or missed recording on notes; no follow-up procedure for this
- ❑ No patient progress notes from patient

SLOW DOWNS IN PRACTICE GROWTH

- ❑ Fear of loss
- ❑ Fear of the unknown
- ❑ Boredom with the passage of time
- ❑ Monotonous repetition
- ❑ Quantity sacrificing quality
- ❑ Referrals taken for granted
- ❑ Dropping out the early things in practice, extras, which made practice initially successful
- ❑ Reduction in personal service
- ❑ Front office procedure problems
- ❑ Personnel slack or overworked

Practitioner and Staff's External Attitude:
- ❑ Practitioner cares, but is't showing it
- ❑ Aloof and apart from those one serves
- ❑ Unconcerned with human relations
- ❑ Indifferent to the need for patient education and client motivation
- ❑ Challenged or insulted by people's questions, objections and procrastinations
- ❑ Unappreciative of the opportunity to serve
- ❑ Resistant to change in the status quo.
- ❑ Entitled to practice success by virtue of professional training and license, but behavior doesn't match the vision.

OTHER PROCEDURES INHIBITING GROWTH AND EXPANSION

Referral Procedure
- ❑ Not asking for referrals from patients or other practitioners
- ❑ In receiving referrals on aconsulting or treating basis from other colleagues, no routine of promptly reporting back
- ❑ Not having a referral base of other practitioners to refer in or out
- ❑ Won't refer patients out.

- Chain reaction of referrals come from low income, trades, poor cash flow sources
- Not asking patients "who referred them" and thus, not following up on the ones referring the patients.
- Not acknowledging those who refer to you.
- No extra special acknowledgment to multiple referring people or practitioners
- Not asking patients to bring family and friends in
- No courtesy consultation cards
- No system for building referrals in your office
- No statistics on the number of incoming personal and professional referrals in your office, patient type, age demographics, etc.
- Taking referrals for granted
- Assistant untrained in dialogue for reinforcing referrals
- Assistant trained but not taking opportunity to ask for referral
- No incentives for referrals, such as free treatment for a referral
- Not focusing on referrals -- 75% of new patients should be from referrals
- No networking with other practitioners in your niche or complementary niche

Education Procedure
- No audiovisual aids, such as verbal and written recommendations, directions, do's and don'ts for care, exercise sheets, pamphlets, models, audiovisual tapes
- Tacky audiovisual aids
- No planned education of patients or community re: your services, their benefits, importance of follow-through care
- No acupuncture health care classes
- No lecture or demonstration in the community with sign-up sheets for consultation

Advertising Procedures
- Investing in advertising without professional ad consultation and advice
- No advertising
- No newspaper column with your picture educating patients about you and acupuncture care
- Ads which don't have what it takes to motivate a reader to action
- Relying primarily on paid advertising for new patients
- Advertising too general, doesn't address your niche, pain, or your specialty
- Expensive advertising, low yield results

- ❑ Sensational or gimmicky advertising
- ❑ Ad too small to be noticed
- ❑ Picture and words don't match. No graphics. Your graphics aren't getting attention.
- ❑ Headline doesn't make you read the ad
- ❑ Nonprofessional ad
- ❑ Good ad, too infreQuent
- ❑ Not using the best space in a publication for a health care ad
- ❑ Over 10% of gross receipts in advertising, established practitioner
- ❑ Over 20% of gross receipts, new practitioners (under 18 months)
- ❑ No reconciliation of cost of advertising
- ❑ Advertising expenses too out of balance with income results

After reviewing this list, look at your practice plan and write down what you intend to do to move to the next stage of your practice success. Comments:

In Sum

You are capable of both surrendering to your destiny – each step along the way – and making things happen. Totally believe in your ability. Trust your intuition. You attract those who respond to your natural way of empowering people, promoting their well-being, nurturing those who have need, and attending to the details of their health care.

Accept yourself and your practice at fact value. Your practice will be unlike any others because it reflects who you are – the whole bag of your godlike qualities and human failings, specific gifts and lessons to learn.

Acknowledge your expertise and competencies as a healer. If there is a question that you have not asked or to which you have been unable to find the answer, do not consider the matter closed. If you have not thought of a problem, or, having thought of it, you have not resolved it, do not think the matter settled. Consult with the experts in areas where you need greater clarity. Your patients will feel you go the extra mile for them. Tell them the truth of what you see. You serve them best by your realness, your honesty, and your deliberate attention to their well-being. If there is a principle which you have been unable to put into practice do not let up. If one person gets there with one try, try ten times. If another succeeds with a hundred tries, make a thousand. Proceeding in this manner, even one who is a bit slow will find the light; even a weak person will find energy.

Take advantage of refining the details of managing your practice. Be aware that your staff is like a backbone and internal organs the body. Take care of your staff, and they will operate your practice smoothly and care for you and your patients well. Patients notice and seem to get well when the office is light, in sync and attention is paid to those fine details - where the reception room is fresh and alive with plants, comfortable furniture, interesting people and literature; where their concerns are heard and researched, appointments and insurance questions and billing are handled clearly – where they see beneficial staff teamwork.

Listen and notice when you need to do your homework. 'Take the time' to reevaluate your practice and your experience. As you go back and look at the exercises in the guide later, you will receive new and affirming answers. Redefine your goals in the light of your expanding vision, and establish a plan to implement those goals. Set guideline times to begin and complete not only the opening of your practice, but times to look at, adjust, refine, and expand it. Readjust your framework as needed so that you don't self-create unnecessary stress. Be present, on purpose and enjoy working your plan! Experience and acknowledge your success.

Trust the process of growth. Your practice will season with time. There are periods of gestation and thrust, plateaus and expansion; smooth sailing and turbulence, shifts and rest. For those of you who experience the fulfillment of flourishing, established practices, you know that holding, attaining and expanding your vision are all part of the process of simply enjoying your creation.

In sum: Rise above the mediocre and acknowledge your center – your source of love and power. Be confident in your ability to start, expand, and sustain your practice. Exercise your humility when you need guidance, and receive it. Consciously radiate caring, clarity and service, and that motivating force to all with whom you come in contact. Love the world as your Self. It is then you may be truly entrusted with all things under the Sun.

From one being to another, I have infinite faith in you.

BIBLIOGRAPHY

Agran, Larry. "How Necessary is a Written Business Partnership Agreement?" *Los Angeles Times Home Magazine*, June 20, 1982

Albrecht, Dr. Karl. *Successful Management by Objectives*. Prentice-Hall, Inc., Englewood Cliffs, New Jersey, 1978.

American Chiropractic Association. *Chiropractic Paraprofessional Manual: Practice Administration and Management*, 1978. (Paraphrased material used bearing author's full responsibility).

American Medical Association. *Physicians' Current Procedural Terminology, CPT*, 1988 edition, Chicago, 1987 - 1996.

Ball, Kurt. *Leasing: Questions and Answers*, Santa Barbara, 1986.

Bandler & Grinder. *Frogs into Princes*. Real People Press, Moab, Utah, 1979.

Bartlett, Pringle & Wolf. *Business Taxes – Tax Information on Federal Withholding & Payroll Taxes*, Santa Barbara, 1987 and Cook, Michael. CPA, *Updated Revisions*, Maui, 1987.

Bass, Steven. *Successful Private Practice*, Pasadena, 1986.

Bass, Steven. *Successful Insurance Reimbursement*, Pasadena, 1987.

Beck, Leif, C. *The Physician's Office*, Princeton, J.J. Excerpta Medica, 1977.

Board of Medical Quality Assurance. Acupuncture Examining Committee. *Laws and Regulations to the Practice of Acupuncture*. State of California Dept. of Consumer Affairs, 1988.

Chan, K.C. Fee Schedule: *Treatment Plan by Visit & by Diagnosis*. San Diego, 1985.

City of Santa Barbara. *Local Business Tax and Permit Licensing.* 1987.

Clydesdale, Joyce. *Clydesdale Institute Practice Manual*, self published.

Department of Consumer Affairs. *Patient's Access to Medical Records: Summary*. Acupuncture Examining Committee, 1985.

Everard/Shilt. *Business Principles & Management.* 7th Edition. by permission of South Western Publishing Co., Cincinnati, Ohio, 1979. Material reviewed and updated by Michael Cook, CPA, Maui, 1987.

Fernandez, Dr. Peter. *Secrets of a Practice Management Consultant.*

Fernandez, Dr. Peter. *How to Start a Profitable Practice from Scratch.* 2nd edition, 1980.

Flamholtz, Eric G. & Randle, Yvonne. *The Inner Game of Management.* American Management Association, New York, 1987.

Holtz, Herman, *The Direct Marketer's Workbook.* John Wiley & Sons, New York, 1986.

Hua, Ellen Kei. *Kung Fu Meditations & Chinese Proverbial Wisdom.* Thor Publishing, Ventura, California, 1981.

Crocker, Charles R., D.C. *Insurance Reporting.* Kingsland, Georgia

Jones, Seymour et al. *The Coopers & Lybrand Guide to Growing Your Business.* Wiley & Sons, New York, 1988.

IRS Publications. *Business Use of the Home.* 1986.

Kamoroff, Bernard, CPA. *Small Time Operator: How to Start Your Own Small `Business, Keep Your Books, Pay Your Taxes and Stay Out of Trouble.* Bell Springs Publishing, Laytonville, 1986.

Kuhns, Dr. Bradley, C.A. *Mind/Body Therapy: Visual, Auditory, Kinesthetic, An Additional Communication Approach for the Counselor.*

Levoy, Robert, P. *The Successful Professional Practice.* Prentice-Hall, Inc. Englewood Cliffs, New Jersey, 1970.

Mackenzie, R. Alec. *The Time Trap.* McGraw-Hill, New York, 1975.

Mancuso, Joseph R. *How to Write a Winning Business Plan.* Prentice-Hall Press, New York, 1985.

Nall, Steven. "The Secret to Increase Growth with Less Stress", *MPI's Dynamic Chiropractic.* (January 1988): 20-21.

Porteous, Brian, D.C. "Marketing", *MPI's Dynamic Chiropractic* (March 1988: 34-35, April 1988, August 1988.

Retzler, Kathryn. *How to Start a Service Business and Make it Succeed.* Scott, Foresman and Company. Glenview, Illinois, 1987.

Resnik, Paul. *The Small Business Bible.* Wiley & Sons, Inc., New York, 1988.

Schwab, Victor. *How to Write a Good Advertisement,* A Short Course in Copywriting. Wilshire Book Company. North Hollywood, California, 1962.

Singer, Dr. David. *Staff Policy.* 1984 revised.

Small Business Administration Pamphlets. "Starting and Managing a Small Business on your Own."

Small Business Administration Pamphlets. "Business Plan for Small Service Firms", Handout: "Financial Factors of Business", "Profit and Loss Statement."

Small Business Administration Pamphlets: "Keeping Records In Small Business."

Small Business Administration Pamphlets: "Buying and Selling a Small Business," "Legal Structures of Business."

The Parker School for Professional Success. *Textbook of Office Procedure and Practice Building for the Chiropractic Profession.* The Parker Chiropractic Research Foundation, Inc. Fort Worth, Texas, 1975.

Whole Health Institute. Elaine Gagne. "Quality Circles and Effectiveness in the Office", *Wellness in Action, 1982.*

Workers' Compensation Labor Board. *Workers' Compensation, RVS Fee Schedule for California.* 1987, 1996.

Workers' Compensation Labor Board. *Workers' Compensation, RVS Fee Schedule for Hawaii.* 1987.

Note:
All attempts have been made to contact all known resources for material contained in this manual in order to credit and clear copyrighted material. Therefore, the author will not be responsible for any written material that bears similarity to other person's written material other than those contacted. To anyone who remains unbeknown and unacknowledged, please contact the author so that you may be acknowledge in future supplements.

OFFICE - NEW PATIENT CPT CODES

99201	LEVEL 1	Hist./Exam Str. Forward Decision.	10 min.
99202	LEVEL 2	Hist./Exam Expanded Decision	20 min.
99203	LEVEL 3	Hist./Exam Detailed Decision.	30 min.
99204	LEVEL 4	Hist./Exam Comprehensive	45 min
99205	LEVEL 5	Hist./Exam High Complexity	60 min.

OFFICE ESTABLISHED PATIENT CPT CODES

99211	LEVEL 1	Exam/Hist. Straight Forward	5 min.
99212	LEVEL 2	Exam/Hist. Expanded	10 min.
99213	LEVEL 3	Exam/Hist. Detailed	15 min.
99214	LEVEL 4	Exam./Hist. Report of Find.	25 min.
99215	LEVEL 5	Exam/Hist. Hi Complex	40 min.

Modifiers for OFFICE VISIT Eval. and Mgmt Codes above:
-21   ADD. time for prolonged evaluation and patient managment
-52   REDUCED FEE modifier (add to existing CPT Service code)

TREATMENT PHYSICAL MEDICINE CPT
Required supervision by MD or DC in some states, unless Lic.Ac. primary care status. Physical Med. Initial 30 min TX to 1 area, except 97799.

MODALITIES

97010	Hot or Cold Packs
97014	Elect. Stim. (unattended)
97024	Diathermy
97026	Infrared
97032	Elect. Stim. Manual (attended procedure) Each 15 min.
97035	Ultrasound each 15 min.
97039	Unlisted modality specify type and time _____

PROCEDURES

97124	Massage Procedure
97139	Unlisted Procedure, specify type and time _____
97140	Manual Therapy techniques (eg mobilization, manipulation, manual lymphatic drainage, manual traction one or more regions each 15 min.
97530	Therapeutic activities, direct (one on one) pt. contact by provider Use of dynamic activities to improve functional performance), each 15 min.
97780	Acupuncture one or more needles without electrical stimulation
97781	Acupuncture one or more needles with electrical stimulation
97799	Unlisted physical medicine/rehabilitaiton service or procedure

Modifiers for PROCEDURE Codes: (add these codes to procedures, ie 97124-22. (See CPT Code Book from the AMA for other modifiers)
-22   ADD. time for unusual procedural service
-52   REDUCED FEE modifier (add to existing Procedure CPT code)

OTHER SPECIAL CATEGORY CPT CODES (See section re: laser)

64550	TNS neuro stim. surgical procedure code
99070	Needles
99070	Supplements (list) Herbs and Nutrition, other
99070	Orthopedic support/ pillows _____
99080	Special Report

CONSULTATION OFFICE CPT
New or Established Patient

99241	Level 1	Limited	15 min.
99242	Level 2	Expanded	30 min.
99243	Level 3	Detailed	40 min.
99244	Level 4	Comprehensive	60 min.
99245	Level 5	Complex (revised)	80 min.

Follow-up visits in consultant's office or other outpatient facility that are initiated by the physician consultant are reported using office visit codes for established patients (99211-99215)

HOME SERVICES CPT

99341-99345	Levels 1-5 New Patient Limited, Expanded, Detailed, Comprehensive, High Complex,
99347-99350	Levels 1-3, and level 5 Estab. Patient Limited, Expanded, Detailed, High Complex

____ STATE AID CODE Acupuncture
____ WORK COMP. RVS CODE Acupuncture

OFFICE - NEW PATIENT CPT CODES

99201	Same
99202	Same
99203	Same
99204	Same
99205	Same

OFFICE - NEW PATIENT CPT CODES

99211	Same
99212	Same
99213	Same
99214	Same
99215	Same

TREATMENT PHYSICAL MEDICINE CPT
Required supervision by MD, or DC some states, unless Lic. Ac. primary care status

MODALITIES

97010	Same
97014	Same
97024	Same
97026	Same
97032	Same
97035	Same
97039	Same

PROCEDURES

97124	Same
97139	Same
97250	Delete, Changed
97530	Same
97780	Same
97781	Same
97799	Same

Modifiers for PROCEDURE Codes

-22	Same
-52	Same

OTHER SPECIAL CATEGORY CPT CODES

64550	Same
99070	Same
99070	Same
99070	Same
99080	Same

INITIAL CONSULTATION (no treatment)
New Patient

99241	Same
99242	Same
99243	Same
99244	Same
99245	Same

Follow-up visits Same

HOME SERVICES CPT

99341-99343	1999 uses basic mgmt coded 5 levels
99351-99353	Deleted

____ Check with your state reg. board for new changes
____ Check with your state reg. board for new changes